HOSPICE AND PALLIATIVE CARE TRAINING FOR PHYSICIANS: A SELF-STUDY PROGRAM

Third Edition

UNIPAC 2

Alleviating Psychological and Spiritual Pain in Patients with Life-Limiting Illness

Holly M. Holmes, MD
University of Texas MD Anderson
 Cancer Center
Houston, TX

Regina Stein, MD
Hematology-Oncology Associates
 of Illinois, LLC
Northwestern University
Chicago, IL

Carol F. Knight, EdM
Knight Consultants
Austin, TX

Reviewed by
Randy S. Hebert, MD MPH
University of Pittsburgh Medical Center
Pittsburgh, PA

Edited by
C. Porter Storey, Jr., MD FACP FAAHPM*
with
Stacie Levine, MD[†]
Joseph W. Shega, MD**

 * *Colorado Permanente Medical Group, Boulder, CO; American Academy of Hospice and Palliative Medicine, Glenview, IL*
 † *University of Chicago, Chicago, IL*
 ** *Northwestern University, Chicago, IL*

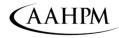
AAHPM

American Academy of Hospice and Palliative Medicine
4700 W. Lake Avenue
Glenview, IL 60025-1485
www.aahpm.org

© 2008 American Academy of Hospice and Palliative Medicine
First edition published 1997
Second edition published 2003

ISBN 978-1-889296-22-7

Contents

Tables

Figures

Acknowledgments

The editors, authors, contributors, and the American Academy of Hospice and Palliative Medicine (AAHPM) are deeply grateful to all who have participated in the development of this component of the *Hospice and Palliative Care Training for Physicians: UNIPAC* self-study program. The expertise of the contributors and reviewers involved in the first, second, and now the third edition of the UNIPACs has greatly improved their value and content. Our special thanks are extended to the original authors of this book, C. Porter Storey, Jr., MD FACP FAAHPM, and Carol F. Knight, EdM, and to the professionals who generously volunteered their time and experience to review this book and test its contents in the field—Ira R. Byock, MD FAAHPM; John W. Finn, MD FAAHPM; Walter B. Forman, MD; Rev. Milton W. Hay, DMin; Gerald H. Holman, MD FAAFP; Rev. Charles Meyer, MDiv MS; Terry C. Muck, PhD; Eli N. Perencevich, DO; Charles G. Sasser, MD; Julia L. Smith, MD; and Bradley Stuart, MD.

Continuing Medical Education

Purpose

A UNIPAC is a packet of information formatted as an independent-study program. It includes learning objectives, a pretest, reading material, clinical situations for demonstrating knowledge application, references, and a posttest. This independent-study program is intended for physicians and physicians in training. It is designed to increase competence in palliative medical interventions for improving a patient's quality of life, particularly as death approaches. Specific, practical information is presented to help physicians assess and manage selected problems. After reading the UNIPAC, physicians are encouraged to seek additional training in hospice and palliative medicine.

Learning Objectives

Upon completion of this continuing medical education (CME) program, a physician should be better able to
- identify common reactions to loss
- use predictors to assess the likelihood of complicated reactions to loss
- use effective interventions to reestablish a patient's sense of purpose
- use effective interventions to enhance a patient's sense of efficacy
- use effective interventions to foster hope
- assess and manage anxiety and depression with pharmacological and nonpharmacological interventions
- differentiate complicated and uncomplicated grief reactions
- assess for spiritual pain and provide effective basic interventions
- involve other team members in alleviating psychological and spiritual pain.

Recommended Procedure

To receive maximum benefit from this UNIPAC, the following procedure is recommended:
- Review the learning objectives.
- Complete the pretest before reading the UNIPAC.
- Study each section and the clinical situations.
- Review the correct responses to the pretest.
- Complete the online posttest by following the instructions listed on page 85 of this book.

Some accrediting organizations may not accept the CME from the third edition of the UNIPAC series if you have already obtained CME for the previous edition of the same UNIPAC. For clarification, please contact your accrediting organization.

Accreditation Statement

The American Academy of Hospice and Palliative Medicine (AAHPM) is accredited by the Accreditation Council for Continuing Medical Education (ACCME) to provide continuing medical education for physicians. AAHPM designates this continuing medical education activity for a maximum of six (6) *AMA PRA Category 1 Credits*™.

Physicians are eligible to receive credit by completing both the online evaluation form and posttest. The Academy will keep a record of *AMA PRA Category 1 Credits*™, and the record will be provided on request; however, physicians are responsible for reporting their own credits when applying for the AMA/PRA or for other certificates or credentials.

Disclosure

In accordance with the Accreditation Council for Continuing Medical Education's Standards for Commercial Support, all CME providers are required to disclose to the activity audience the relevant financial relationships of the planners, teachers, and authors involved in the development of CME content. An individual has a relevant financial relationship if he or she has a financial relationship in any amount occurring in the last 12 months with a commercial interest whose products or services are discussed in the CME activity content over which the individual has control. AAHPM requires that all relevant financial relationships be resolved before planning or participating in the activity.

Holly Holmes, MD, has disclosed no relevant financial relationships. **Regina Stein, MD,** has disclosed no relevant financial relationships. **Carol F. Knight, EdM,** has disclosed no relevant financial relationships. **Randy S. Hebert, MD MPH,** has disclosed no relevant financial relationships. **C. Porter Storey, Jr., MD FACP FAAHPM,** has disclosed no relevant financial relationships. **Stacie Levine, MD,** has disclosed no relevant financial relationships. **Joseph W. Shega, MD,** has disclosed no relevant financial relationships.

Review and Revision

This book was reviewed by AAHPM's UNIPAC Review Task Force and reapproved by the American Academy of Hospice and Palliative Medicine's board of directors.

Term of Offering

The release date for the third edition of this UNIPAC is May 31, 2008, and the expiration date is December 31, 2011. Final date to request credit is December 31, 2011.

Posttest Pass Rate

The posttest pass rate is 75%.

Additional Information

Additional information is available from the American Academy of Hospice and Palliative Medicine, where staff can direct you to physicians specializing in end-of-life care.

This independent-study program was originally supported in part by federal funds from the National Cancer Institute's Cancer Education Grant Program, Grant CA66771. The third edition of the Hospice and Palliative Care Training for Physicians: UNIPAC *self-study program received no federal or commercial financial support.*

Pretest

Before proceeding, please complete the following multiple-choice questions. The answers are listed on page 83 of this book.

1. Which of the following interventions is *least* likely to relieve the suffering associated with serious or life-threatening illness?
   A. Providing a calm and empathetic presence
   B. Ordering diagnostic tests to locate the primary site of a cancer
   C. Communicating effectively
   D. Setting short-term, attainable goals

2. Which of the following statements about pain is true?
   A. Physical pain is never the most important contributor to suffering.
   B. Total pain refers to the physical, psychological, spiritual, and social pain experienced by dying patients.
   C. The distress associated with spiritual pain rarely exacerbates physical symptoms.
   D. Well-controlled physical symptoms interfere with a patient's ability to interact with loved ones.

3. Which of the following actions is most likely to help physicians cope with the stresses associated with caring for dying patients?
   A. Never acknowledge periodic feelings of grief, helplessness, and fear.
   B. Let go of attachments to family and outside interests and concentrate on professional activities.
   C. Exercise, rest, and practice a spiritual discipline.
   D. Refuse to let others meddle in the management of difficult cases.

4. Which of the following reactions to a spouse's death is *least* expected?
   A. Periods of breathlessness or fatigue
   B. Brief visual and auditory hallucinations of the deceased
   C. Periodic thoughts of not wanting to go on living
   D. Calm acceptance of the death within a week

5. Which of the following is *least* likely to predict a person's reaction to a traumatic loss?
   A. The nature of the person's attachment to the deceased
   B. Personality factors such as a tendency to depression
   C. Previous responses to expected and timely losses
   D. Presence of supportive networks such as family, church, or social groups

6. Which of the following statements about grief is *least* likely to be true?
   A. Reactions to a death are affected by the bereaved person's attachment to the deceased.
   B. Ambivalent relationships are unrelated to complicated grief.
   C. Prolonged yearning and anger are common reactions to the death of a child.
   D. Protracted disorganization is a common reaction to the death of a spouse.

7. Which of the following is *least* likely to characterize a successful adaptation to loss?
   A. Rebuilding assumptions about the world and self
   B. Making sense of the loss by reconstructing meaning
   C. Concentrating on work-related activities and ignoring the loss
   D. Letting go of previous roles that can no longer be maintained

8. Which of the following is the *least* important aspect of the developmental tasks of the dying?
   A. Completing all unfinished business before death occurs
   B. Developing an enlarged and renewed sense of personhood and meaning
   C. Bringing as much closure as possible to personal and community relationships
   D. Accepting increased dependency

9. Which of the following statements about meaning is true?
   A. The need for meaning is only determined by culture.
   B. Common sources of meaning include family, work, and religious or political affiliations.
   C. Sources of meaning are unlikely to change over the course of a lifetime.
   D. Most people can identify one unifying meaning for their lives.

10. Which of the following statements about suffering is true?
    A. Suffering does not occur in the absence of physical pain.
    B. Suffering is rarely related to thoughts about the future.
    C. Suffering results from losses that threaten a person's entire sense of self.
    D. Suffering increases when the integrity of personhood is restored by reestablishing meaning and hope.

11. When physical pain contributes to suffering, which of the following interventions is most likely to be helpful?
    A. Challenge the validity of the patient's experience of pain.
    B. Avoid upsetting the patient with information about the source of pain, even when requested.
    C. Demonstrate that pain can be controlled with adequate dosages of appropriate medications.
    D. Help patients reframe the meaning of comfort.

12. Which of the following statements about suffering is true?
    A. Suffering is unrelated to role expectations.
    B. In most cases, sources of suffering can be identified and alleviated.
    C. Suffering is unrelated to future events; it focuses on the present.
    D. Suffering rarely results in a powerful need to make sense of events.

13. Which of the following statements is *least* likely to be true?
    A. Suffering provides a powerful impetus for reconstructing meaning.
    B. A competent physician can generally cure all aspects of a patient's suffering.
    C. The meanings attached to specific events can cause suffering.
    D. With caring intervention, suffering can lead to an enlarged sense of self.

14. Which of the following statements about assessing for psychological and spiritual pain is most likely to be true?
    A. Patients tend to report what they believe the physician is least interested in hearing.
    B. To effectively assess for the presence of total pain, clinicians should avoid asking specific questions about psychological and spiritual issues.
    C. Ongoing assessment is important because patients may be unable or unwilling to discuss such issues during the first interview.
    D. During the first interview, patients are more likely to discuss spiritual pain than physical pain.

15. Which of the following statements is *least* likely to be true?
    A. Interventions to relieve suffering should focus on general issues instead of specific problems.
    B. When a patient is suffering, relieving distressing physical symptoms should be the first step.
    C. Effective interventions to relieve suffering utilize the skills of the entire interdisciplinary team.
    D. Effective interventions to relieve suffering enhance a patient's search for a renewed sense of meaning, hope, purpose, value, efficacy, and self-worth.

16. Which of the following statements about communication is most likely to be true?
    A. Good communication contributes to suffering by exacerbating the patient's and family's sense of isolation, helplessness, and anxiety.
    B. Information should not be repeated several times because stress interferes with the ability to hear and retain information.
    C. Patients should never be given complete information about their illness and prognosis.
    D. Art, literature, and music can help patients give voice to their suffering.

17. Which of these statements about empathetic presence is most likely to be true?
    A. Empathetic presence is most important after patients have died.
    B. The body language that best expresses empathetic presence is sitting near the patient's bedside.
    C. Empathetic presence often increases patient and family anxiety.
    D. Empathetic presence does not help alleviate the patient's fears about the future.

18. Which of the following interventions is most likely to help a patient with serious or life-threatening illness who is searching for meaning?
    A. Challenge the difficulty of maintaining a sense of purpose.
    B. Concentrate on identifying several purposes that have provided other patients with meaning over the course of their lifetimes.
    C. Help patients find a purpose in "being" rather than "doing."
    D. Discourage patients from talking about the past and help them focus on the present and future.

19. Which of the following actions is *least* likely to help patients reestablish a sense of value, let go of unfinished business, and accept forgiveness?
    A. Acknowledge the difficulty of maintaining a sense of value.
    B. Discourage a patient from requesting religious rituals such as confession or absolution from sin.
    C. Help patients recognize themes of positive value in their life stories.
    D. Help patients find a higher level of meaning in their actions.

20. Which of the following measures is most likely to help patients reestablish a sense of efficacy?
    A. Excuse patients from meetings involving treatment decisions.
    B. Teach patients coping strategies such as relaxation, reframing, and assertiveness.
    C. Encourage patients to accept the physician's explanation of events instead of developing their own.
    D. Help patients avoid explanations that provide only individual meaning for them.

21. Which of the following measures is *least* likely to help patients reestablish a sense of self-worth?
    A. Avoid specific discussions about how the illness is affecting the patient's sense of self-worth.
    B. Listen to the patient's life story.
    C. Validate the patient's experiences with the illness.
    D. Make observations that help patients recognize meaning in their lives.

22. Which of the following statements about hope is true?
    A. Few patients experience a sense of hope during a terminal illness.
    B. For terminally ill patients, the focus of hope is always on finding a cure.
    C. Strategies for maintaining hope are unlike those for alleviating suffering.
    D. A supportive relationship with a physician can help patients maintain hope.

23. When death is near, and severe physical or spiritual pain cannot be relieved by any other means, which of the following interventions is *least* likely to be effective?
    A. Phenobarbital, 130 mg SC hourly until calm, and then by SC infusion (600-1,200 mg/day)
    B. Thiopental, 20 mg to 200 mg hourly continuous IV infusion titrated to relief
    C. Methohexital sodium, continuous IV infusion titrated to relief
    D. Amitriptyline, 20 mg to 30 mg IM four times a day and as needed

24. In the terminally ill population, which of the following is *least* likely to cause anxiety?
    A. Medical complications such as uncontrolled pain, delirium, and sepsis
    B. Biographical factors such as age and race
    C. Abrupt withdrawal from certain medications
    D. Psychological and social factors such as isolation, guilt, and denial

25. When managing anxiety for patients with serious or life-limiting illness, which of the following should receive *least* consideration?
    A. The patient's subjective level of distress
    B. The patient's response to supportive counseling, education, and caring human contact
    C. Involving a social worker and chaplain
    D. Initiating long-term psychoanalysis to resolve deep-seated conflicts occurring during infancy

26. For patients with serious or life-limiting illness, which of the following pharmacologic interventions for anxiety is *least* likely to be effective?

    A. Lorazepam, 0.5 mg to 1.0 mg PO or SL twice a day
    B. Propranolol, 50 mg four times a day
    C. Alprazolam, 0.25 mg to 0.5 mg PO four times a day
    D. Thioridazine, 25 mg to 100 mg PO two to four times a day

27. For patients with serious or life-limiting illness, which of the following is the most common symptom of depression?

    A. Relief from suicidal ideation
    B. Anorexia, fatigue, and sleep difficulties
    C. Pervasive despondency and despair
    D. A renewed sense of meaning and worth

28. Which of the following is *least* likely to be the best treatment for depression in patients with serious or life-limiting illness?

    A. Sertraline, 50 mg once a day for a depressed patient who has insomnia
    B. Gabapentin, 300 mg to 900 mg once a day for a depressed patient with neuropathic pain
    C. Alprazolam, 0.25 mg twice a day for a depressed patient with mixed anxiety and depression
    D. Methylphenidate, 10 mg at 8 am and again at noon for a depressed patient with vegetative symptoms

29. When caring for patients with serious or life-limiting illness who are contemplating suicide, which of the following interventions is *least* likely to be helpful?

    A. Relieve uncontrolled physical symptoms and discontinue treatments (eg, artificial nutrition) that no longer meet their therapeutic goals.
    B. Provide supportive counseling.
    C. Arrange for psychiatric hospitalization.
    D. Involve team members with specialized training in alleviating spiritual and psychological pain.

30. Which of the following symptoms is *least* likely to indicate that the grief is complicated?

    A. Periods of sadness and disorientation that continue for longer than 18 months after the sudden death of a spouse
    B. Levels of depression, anger, and guilt that remain unchanged for months or years after a loss
    C. Suppressed or inhibited expressions of grief
    D. Unexplained chronic disabling physical symptoms that occur after the death of a loved one

31. Which of the following interventions is *least* likely to prevent complicated grief?

    A. Normalize grief by providing information about common reactions to loss.
    B. Suggest that the bereaved person soon find activities that suppress anxiety and depressive symptoms.
    C. Refer the bereaved person to a grief therapist and appropriate support groups.
    D. Help the bereaved person identify losses and express grief.

32. Which of the following statements is *least* likely to be true?

   A. Spirituality is concerned with ultimate issues such as an individual's relationship with the deepest self and the mysteries of life and death.

   B. Religions are organized systems of belief that address universal spiritual questions and offer frameworks of meaning that can be used for making sense of existence.

   C. Religious beliefs and practices can be powerful sources of inspiration and comfort for many people and sources of distress and anxiety for others.

   D. People who attend church regularly are less likely to suffer from spiritual pain than those who describe themselves as agnostic or atheist.

33. Which of the following statements is *least* likely to be true?

   A. Patients rarely voice spiritual concerns until distressing physical symptoms are alleviated.

   B. Spiritual pain can be difficult to assess because it shares the following features with depression: pervasive guilt, hopelessness, and worthlessness.

   C. During the initial assessment process it is important to avoid asking specific questions about spiritual pain, guilt, or fear.

   D. In many cases patients are willing to discuss spiritual issues as long as physicians exhibit real interest, demonstrate knowledge of spiritual concerns, and show nonjudgmental respect for various religious and spiritual beliefs.

34. Which of the following statements is most likely to be true?

   A. Most spiritual pain is too deep seated to be addressed during the course of a terminal illness.

   B. Clinicians should use religious terminology and reassure patients that their illness is "God's will."

   C. Most patients and families derive comfort from exploring spiritual issues, even though universally accepted answers do not exist.

   D. Clinicians should avoid issues of guilt and remorse and encourage patients to concentrate on positive thoughts and getting well.

35. Which of the following statements is most likely to be true?

   A. Spiritual pain can sometimes be alleviated with a supportive presence and exploration of issues such as guilt, blame, remorse, forgiveness, and reconciliation.

   B. Inner resources can be strengthened with devotional practices such as meditation, reading scriptures, and prayer.

   C. Past religious beliefs usually provide adequate spiritual support during a terminal illness.

   D. As death approaches there is little benefit in helping patients observe religious practices.

36. Which of the following statements is most likely to be *false*?

   A. Jewish and Islamic customs discourage cremation.

   B. Hindu and Buddhist customs encourage cremation.

   C. Christians place more emphasis on modesty than do most Hindus or Buddhists.

   D. Hindus and Buddhists are often vegetarians.

37. Which of the following statements is *least* likely to be true?
    A. The spiritual practice of daily bathing in running water is more important for Hindus and Muslims than for Christians.
    B. Nonmuslim caregivers should put on rubber gloves before touching the corpse of a Muslim patient and should turn the corpse's head toward the right.
    C. Observing religious traditions and participating in family-oriented religious rituals are particularly important for followers of Judaism.
    D. Following dietary laws is more important for Christians than for Hindus, Buddhists, Jews, or Muslims.

Suffering and Total Pain

Who is there in all the world who listens to us? Here I am—this is me in my nakedness, with my wounds, my secret grief, my despair, my betrayal, my pain which I can't express, my terror, my abandonment. Oh, listen to me for a day, an hour, a moment, lest I expire in my terrible wilderness, my lonely silence. Oh God, is there no one to listen?[1]

—SENECA

Many people suffer terribly from advanced cancer and other chronic diseases.[2,3] Almost 50% of conscious, hospitalized patients experience serious pain in the days before death.[4] Nonphysical causes of suffering in terminal illness have not been studied as extensively as physical causes. Although significant advances have been made in the alleviation of pain and other symptoms caused by advanced illness, the thorough treatment of suffering must incorporate assessment and treatment of psychological, social, and existential or spiritual aspects of suffering.[5]

It may become difficult to distinguish whether suffering at the end of life is caused by physical symptoms or psychosocial or spiritual issues.[6] Unrelieved suffering is associated with a poor quality of life[5] and destroys a patient's opportunity for satisfaction and growth during the final days of life.[7]

A Definition of Suffering

In his book *The Nature of Suffering and the Goals of Medicine*, Eric Cassell defines suffering as a state of severe distress associated with events that threaten the intactness of personhood or the interconnected physical, social, spiritual, and psychological aspects of self.[8] Important predictors of suffering include regret for past events, current marital problems, little social support, and a pessimistic attitude.[9] Suffering may be an unbearable state experienced as

- a split between the self and the now malfunctioning body
- a loss of self-identity[10]
- a sense of isolation from the human community
- fear about continued or recurring physical or psychological pain[8]
- a sense of separation from transcendent truth.[11]

Medicine and the Deconstruction of Suffering

Although the experience of suffering is extremely complex, the medical profession tends to deconstruct it and focus on its simplest component—physical distress, which physicians can usually control. Deconstructing suffering offers a false sense of control; it not only distances physicians from a patient's deeply troubling distress, but it also encourages both physicians and patients to suppress their awareness of the larger meanings of suffering.[12,13]

The long-term results of this narrow focus include

- objectification of suffering as represented by physical pain and symptoms only
- devaluation of important components of the patient's personhood
- excessive reliance on data from diagnostic procedures rather than a patient's report of symptoms
- loss of empathetic communication skills, focusing on the body rather than the whole person.

A central purpose of palliative medicine is to provide comfort and improve quality of life. Providing comfort must include not only the effective management of physical suffering but also the psychosocial, existential, and spiritual aspects of suffering. Physicians experienced in hospice and palliative medicine can effectively manage the difficult physical symptoms that often accompany the dying process, but the management of suffering, with its complex psychological and spiritual components, occasionally tests the limits of even the most experienced clinician.[14] Unless physicians understand the psychological and spiritual pain that often accompany dying and bereavement and the multifaceted nature of loss and suffering, their interventions may not only fail to relieve suffering, they may also become sources of additional suffering.[8]

The Concept of Total Pain

Dr. Cicely Saunders developed the concept of total pain to describe the intense suffering frequently experienced by dying patients and their family members as they traverse the continuum of living the last months of life, dying, death, and bereavement.[15]

Total pain consists of at least four contributors:
- physical pain
- social pain
- psychological pain
- spiritual pain.

The four contributors to total pain, or suffering, are interactive. Unrelieved physical symptoms contribute to emotional and spiritual pain by narrowing the patient's focus and interfering with the ability to interact with loved ones and resolve death-related psychological and spiritual concerns. The deep distress caused by spiritual, psychological, and social pain aggravates the distress caused by physical pain and other symptoms such as nausea and dyspnea. **Table 1** lists common contributors to total pain.

Table 1. Contributors to Total Pain
Uncontrolled pain and other distressing physical symptoms
Major depression
Loss of hope and meaning
Loss of important roles in life
Terror related to approaching death
Severe existential distress
Inability to trust others
Unresolved guilt
Financial distress
Family conflicts
Deep wounds from childhood abuse, neglect, or abandonment

Physical Pain and Suffering

Many physicians use the words pain and suffering interchangeably even when referring only to physical pain; however, physical pain and suffering are not the same.[16] A patient's suffering may not be related to the primary symptoms being treated by physicians.[17] Physical pain may be a major component of suffering, but suffering encompasses much more than physical distress and often occurs in the absence of physical pain. Distinguishing between physical pain and suffering (total pain) is clinically important because effective management often requires different interventions.[17]

Even physical sensations of pain can have different meanings; they may be interpreted as acceptable in some contexts and intolerable in others. The pain of childbirth is usually acceptable because it is frequently associated with hope and new life. However, the physical pain associated with terminal illness is more difficult to bear because it may be unrelenting and is often associated with shattered assumptions, terrible losses, and confrontation with the unknown. Any event can support different meanings, depending on its context, individual associations, and cultural expectations.[12]

Table 2 describes situations in which suffering is related to physical pain and suggests interventions.

Assessment of Suffering

As with physical pain, effective interventions for psychological, social, and spiritual pain depend on accurate assessments of their presence and severity. The most effective method of assessment is engaging patients in meaningful dialogue and then carefully asking about the presence of psychological, social, and spiritual concerns. When assessing for total pain, it is important to normalize its presence by commenting on frequent occurrence during any illness, particularly during profound illness. A helpful way to initially assess suffering is to ask a simple, open-ended question such as, "In what way are you suffering?"[17] The following are examples of additional questions to elicit relevant information[18]:

- Most people find that a serious illness affects their lives in unexpected ways. What are some of the ways this illness is affecting your life?

Table 2. Suffering Related to Physical Pain: Situations and Interventions

Situation	Intervention to Relieve Suffering
The physician does not validate the presence or extent of pain.	Validate the presence and extent of pain.
Patients distrust their own perceptions because other people will not accept the presence of chronic, unexplained pain.	
The pain is so severe it overwhelms the patient's ability to focus on anything else.	Demonstrate that pain can be adequately alleviated.
The patient does not believe the pain can be controlled.	
The pain is chronic and seemingly endless.	
The source of the pain is unknown.	Explain the source of the pain to the patient. If the source is unknown, continue to validate its presence.
The meaning of the pain is dire.	Help patients see other meanings for pain. When patients incorrectly believe that increased pain means they are going to die very soon, explain other likely meanings. Encourage and listen to the patient's expressions of fear.

- What are some of your main concerns, worries, and fears about the future?
- How has this illness affected you physically? Emotionally? Spiritually?
- Have you been sad? Frightened?
- What are some of the main problems you are facing now?
- How has this illness affected your relationships with your family? Your friends? Your financial situation?
- What do you miss most as a result of this illness?
- How well do you think you are functioning?
- Do you think about what caused your illness? What are some of your ideas?
- Is something bothering you that you are uncomfortable discussing?
- What are some of the things you wish you could talk about? Who do you wish you could talk to?
- What are some of your family's biggest concerns, worries, or fears? How do you deal with their concerns?
- In the past, what has given you the strength to cope with difficult situations?
- Do you have spiritual or religious beliefs that will influence your decisions about medical care?

Ongoing assessment is vital. The components of total pain are often so interconnected that differentiating them during an initial interview may be almost impossible. Additionally, most patients focus on physical problems during the first interview and may be unable or unwilling to discuss sources of psychological, social, and spiritual pain. **Table 3** describes basic guidelines to follow when assessing for psychological and spiritual pain.

Table 3. Total Pain: Basic Assessment Guidelines

Suspect Total Pain

The index of suspicion for the presence of total pain should be high and should increase when the following occur:

- The patient's physical symptoms are unexplainable and do not respond to usually effective interventions.
- The patient's emotional responses seem out of proportion to the loss.
- Concordance with treatments is erratic.

Establish a Conducive Atmosphere

- Establish a comfortable and unhurried atmosphere.
- Show concern for nonphysical sources of pain.

Express Interest and Ask Specific Questions

- Ask specific questions about psychological, social, and spiritual concerns.
- Be aware that patients often give the following factors stronger importance ratings than do physicians:
  - making funeral arrangements
  - not being a burden to others
  - helping others
  - coming to peace with God
  - being mentally aware.

Listen for Broader Meanings

- Avoid deconstructing an illness (separating it into discrete, smaller parts) when assessing for total pain.
- Assessments should include specific questions designed to elicit a patient's feelings and thoughts about the broader meanings of the illness and the illness's affects on the patient's entire life.

The Physician's Role

Roles of Physicians and Team Members

Effective palliative medicine depends on the skills and resources of an interdisciplinary healthcare team. To help relieve suffering and control physical symptoms, physicians must have some understanding of the psychological and spiritual components of suffering so they can provide basic interventions to help relieve total pain. This includes

- knowing how to recognize the presence of spiritual and psychosocial pain
- involving members of an interdisciplinary team to thoroughly address the different components of suffering
- remaining present and lending strength and support as patients and their caregivers cope with the psychological and spiritual concerns that commonly occur during the process of dying[19]
- supporting patients in their search for a renewed sense of purpose, value, efficacy, and self-worth within their own frameworks of meaning
- recognizing that the physician's job is not to provide all of the answers as much as to show commitment.[20]

Physicians can best alleviate a patient's psychological and spiritual pain by relinquishing their own need to provide all of the answers. Instead, they can join patients and family members in contemplating the profound questions and ultimate mysteries that surround life and death. In many cases empathetic listening is the most therapeutic intervention physicians can offer. This can be a difficult concept for many physicians, who often feel tremendous pressure from themselves and their patients and families to "fix" any discomfort.

Patient's View of the Physician's Role

Most patients believe physicians have a duty to help relieve their suffering regardless of its cause. Patients want physicians to care about them as people, treat them as whole persons, and know what they value. Patients also want their physicians to treat them with dignity and respect and to view them as human beings apart from their illnesses. Finally, patients want their physicians to include them in decision making, control their pain and other symptoms, help them prepare for death, help them achieve a sense of completion, and help alleviate their suffering.[21] (For more specific information on the role of physicians in hospice and palliative care, see UNIPAC 5.)

Communication Barriers in Hospice and Palliative Care

Many barriers prevent optimal assessment and alleviation of suffering. Some patients may have limitations specific to their disease that prevent effective communication, and others may have delirium or other causes of impaired cognition. For example, patients with advanced dementia may not be able to verbally report symptoms; in these cases specialized assessments using nonverbal pain and symptom indicators are necessary.[22] As most illnesses progress, patients are less likely to be able to communicate. In a retrospective study, the prevalence of cancer patients who could communicate in a complex manner in the last 5- , 3- , and 1-day period before death was 43%, 28%, and 13%, respectively.[23]

Alleviating Suffering

During the final phases of a patient's terminal illness, physicians are faced with brief but highly significant opportunities to help patients and families adapt to loss and alleviate their psychological, social, and spiritual distress.[14] In many cases, instead of additional diagnostic tests, medications, or procedures, the five basic interventions listed in **Table 4** are likely to alleviate suffering experienced by patients and their family members.

Fostering Hope

Herth defined hope as "an inner power directed toward enrichment of being."[25] Hope is closely associated with meaning and purpose for patients with advanced illness.[6] Fostering hope is an important way for the interdisciplinary palliative care team to appreciate a

Table 4. Five Basic Hospice and Palliative Care Interventions

Control Pain and Other Distressing Physical Symptoms

Initially consider that distress is caused by uncontrolled physical symptoms (eg, pain, nausea, dyspnea). See UNIPAC 3.
- Use gentle, reassuring touch coupled with scrupulous attention to the details of physical care and symptom relief, especially when patients have difficulty communicating.
- When death is near continue providing excellent symptom control and, if necessary, offer sedation when severe distress cannot be relieved by any other means.

Alleviate Psychosocial Problems

Problems such as loneliness, financial concerns, or the need to arrange care for young children require skillful and ongoing intervention by an entire interdisciplinary team.
- Encourage patients to tell their life stories so biography can be used to identify themes of purpose and value in their lives.
- Focus on specific problems and mobilizing family and community resources.
- Help patients and families let go of previous roles and expectations that interfere with psychological and spiritual healing so they can open up to a new sense of wholeness.

Communicate Effectively

Honest, compassionate, ongoing communication is an essential component of hospice and palliative medicine. Information should be repeated as often as necessary. Physicians can improve a patient's ability to hear what is being said by controlling distressing symptoms, building a therapeutic relationship, and addressing sources of stress.
- Utilize an interdisciplinary team of healthcare professionals.
- Help patients communicate their suffering through biography, art, music, story, and poetry.

Provide Empathic Presence
- Create an atmosphere in which patients and family members feel free to question, examine issues, explore solutions, laugh, cry, and voice their deepest concerns without fear of rejection, isolation, or abandonment.
- Use empathetic body language, including a relaxed presence, sitting down so the physician's eyes are on the same level as the patient's, and sitting as close as the patient desires.
- Remain present when the patient's suffering evokes the physician's own fears and insecurities, and resist the almost-irresistible need to "do something" when listening is the more appropriate action.
- Use the resources of an interdisciplinary team.
- Remain centered and "take the heat" when a patient's and family's suffering manifests as anger, fear, and lack of trust.
- Arrange for meaningful religious sacraments and rituals as desired by the patient.

Foster Hope

The focus of hope changes over the course of illness, from an initial desire for cure and complete recovery to a desire for more intangible states, such as inner peace.
- Use specific hope-enhancing strategies, such as those listed in Table 5.
- Set specific, attainable short-term goals.
- Enhance a patient's sense of hope by involving them in creative arts projects.[24]

patient's values, goals, understanding of their illness, and wishes for the future.[26]

Table 5 lists commonly expressed hopes of dying patients. A simple method to elicit a patient's hopes is to ask, "What do you hope for?" The Herth Hope Index© shown in **Table 6** provides a numerical assessment of hope that may provide a comparison over time.

Loss of hope is an important indicator for suicidal tendency and depression. In a study of terminally ill patients, 37% expressed hopelessness, and patients with hopelessness were more likely to be depressed and to wish for an early death.[6] Hopelessness is part of the "demoralization syndrome," as defined by Kissane,[27] which includes hopelessness, helplessness, loss of coping ability, and lack of social support.

Table 5. Hopes Expressed by Dying Patients[25]

I hope a cure is possible and I will feel better soon.

I hope I will still have pleasurable experiences in my life.

I hope people will deal with me honestly.

I hope people will recognize there are times when I don't want to talk about dying.

I hope treatments will be explained and I will be included in treatment decisions.

I hope my life has meaning.

I hope I can still meet some of the goals that are important to me.

I hope I can get help with the practical things I need to do before I die.

I hope someone will listen to my fears and help me face them.

I hope I will be remembered fondly by my family and friends.

Table 6. Herth Hope Index©

Listed below are a number of statements. Read each statement and place an X in the box that describes how much you agree with that statement right now.

	Strongly Disagree	Disagree	Agree	Strongly Agree
1. I have a positive outlook toward life.				
2. I have short- and/or long-range goals.				
3. I feel all alone.				
4. I can see possibilities in the midst of difficulties.				
5. I have faith that gives me comfort.				
6. I feel scared about my future.				
7. I can recall happy/joyful times.				
8. I have deep inner strength.				
9. I am able to give and receive caring/love.				
10. I have a sense of direction.				
11. I believe that each day has potential.				
12. I feel my life has value and worth.				

Scoring
- All items except items 3 and 6 are scored as follows: Strongly Disagree = 1; Disagree = 2; Agree = 3; Strongly Agree = 4
- Items 3 and 6 are reverse scored as follows: Strongly Disagree = 4; Disagree = 3; Agree = 2; Strongly Agree = 1

No specific score indicates whether a person has adequate hope. However, comparing a patient's responses over time can reveal important information. Discussing the results of each completed index provides an opportunity for professional caregivers to gently probe selected issues with patients and discuss possible interventions, including reframing hope during the course of a terminal illness.

The Herth Hope Index© and scoring instructions must be obtained directly from KA Herth. From Herth K. Abbreviated instrument to measure hope: development and psychometric evaluation. J Adv Nurs. 1992;17:1251-1259. © 1989 Kaye Herth. Reprinted with permission.

The demoralization syndrome is associated with chronic illnesses, disability, disfigurement, fear of loss of dignity, increased social isolation, and increased dependence on others.[6] Physicians and palliative care providers can foster hope by being present, giving information to patients and families, and demonstrating a caring attitude to the patient and family.[24] Specific interventions to foster hope are listed in **Table 7.**

Specific Strategies to Relieve Suffering

Not all strategies for alleviating suffering will be appropriate for every patient. The basis of most treatment for suffering, however, is supportive-expressive therapy, in which the palliative care team accepts and respects the patient, sincerely listens and pays attention to the patient, encourages expression, and reassures the patient that his or her feelings are normal. Some forms of suffering may respond better to other more specific strategies. For example, patients with anxiety may respond to a more comfortable environment, art therapy, relaxation therapy, and the alleviation of physical symptoms. Patients who are suffering because of increased dependency may benefit from meaning-centered therapy, in which life values and life story are explored.[28]

The Dying Process

Before the advent of antibiotics, the process of dying often occurred over the course of days or weeks. As chronic illnesses have become the leading causes of death, however, the process of dying has grown to the extent that it is now recognized as an additional stage of life, like the stages of childhood, adolescence, and adulthood. However, despite the fact that 78% of people in the United States now live past their 65th birthday, and more than three-quarters of them will contend with cancer, stroke, heart disease, obstructive lung disease, or dementia during their last year of life,[29] society continues to struggle with the challenging task of developing culturally meaningful roles and rituals for this newly recognized stage of life.[30]

Palliative care practitioners strive to help patients and families achieve a "good death." The basic characteristics of a good death include reducing internal conflicts, sustaining a patient's sense of identity, maintaining or enhancing existing relationships, and setting limited but

---

Table 7. Strategies That Foster Hope in Patients, Families, and Medical Staff[25]

Provide Comfort and Relieve Suffering
- Effectively control pain and other distressing symptoms (see UNIPAC 3 and UNIPAC 4).
- Acknowledge and address all causes of suffering.

Develop Caring Relationships

Set Attainable Goals and Involve Patients in Decision Making
- Recognize the small joys of the present.
- Develop a sense of purpose or direction that fosters a sense of meaning in life.
- Redefine aims as needed. As physical deterioration becomes more evident, the patient's goals are likely to gradually change from accomplishing specific tangible goals to more global goals that include hopes for the well-being of other people and a sense of "being" rather than "having" or "doing" that includes hope for such things as serenity, inner peace, and eternal rest or life.

Support Spirituality
Regardless of specific religious beliefs, a spiritual foundation can provide a sense of meaning and security that transcends human explanation. Patients and others note that personal attributes such as determination, courage, and serenity have helped them maintain hope.
- Support the use of meaningful religious rites and rituals when requested.
- Identify valued personal attributes and affirm the patient's worth.
- Treat people as dignified, worthwhile human beings.

When Appropriate, Use Light-Hearted Humor
Humor and light-heartedness, when appropriate, can provide a sense of release from thoughts and fears about the disease and can bring joy and hope to a darkened room. Family members may need to be reminded that laughter can be very helpful. For more information on the appropriate use of humor, see UNIPAC 5.

Reminisce About Life and Emphasize Uplifting Memories
Recalling pleasant moments by sharing happy stories, looking at photo albums, and reminiscing about significant events such as the birth of a child can help to maintain hope.

---

reasonable goals. Dying patients are most concerned with alleviating pain and other symptoms, avoiding a prolonged dying process, maintaining a sense of control, relieving burdens of others, and strengthening relationships with loved ones.[6]

Table 8 describes the developmental tasks of dying. These include achieving a sense of completion, relief, and personal growth during the final months and weeks of life. When these tasks are accompanied by personally meaningful rituals, they are likely to enhance the patient's, family's, and clinician's sense of purpose. These rituals are also likely to diminish the patient's spiritual and emotional pain.[31]

Table 8. Developmental Tasks of Dying Patients[31]

Develop a Renewed Sense of Personhood and Meaning

Find meanings in life through life review and personal narrative.

Develop a sense of worthiness, both in the past and in the current situation.

Learn to accept love and caring from other people.

Bring Closure to Personal and Community Relationships

Say goodbye to family members and friends with expressions of regret, gratitude, appreciation, and affection.

Ask for and grant forgiveness to estranged friends and family members so that reconciliation can occur.

Say good-bye to community relationships (employment, civic, and religious organizations) with expressions of regret, gratitude, forgiveness, and appreciation.

Bring Closure to Worldly Affairs

Arrange for the transfer of fiscal, legal, and social responsibilities.

Accept the Finality of Life and Surrender to the Transcendent

Express the depth of personal tragedy that dying may represent and acknowledge the totality of personal loss.

Withdraw from the world and accept increased dependency.

Develop a sense of awe and accept the seeming chaos that can prefigure transcendence.

Some people mistakenly believe that bringing closure to personal or general affairs means completing all the unfinished business of a person's lifetime. Before dying, it is unlikely that a patient will have the ability, time, or energy to engage in long discussions of every past difficulty, tie up all the loose ends of their entire life, or achieve reconciliation with every estranged family member or friend. Instead of encouraging patients to attempt such energetic tasks, physicians should reassure patients that unfinished business is part of the fabric of life and bringing closure to relationships often means focusing on expressing love and asking for and granting forgiveness.[32]

A surprising number of terminally ill patients transcend suffering by viewing their impending death as an opportunity to open up to a larger sense of connectedness and meaning. The ability to adapt and find meaning within the context of a terminal illness offers profound opportunities for society and physicians to learn more about effective interventions for alleviating suffering.

Dignity

Dignity has been described as "deserving honor, respect, or esteem."[6] A person's sense of dignity may be a very personal and transient quality that is highly dependent on values, meanings, goals, and current circumstances. The loss of dignity, particularly in chronic, debilitating, or terminal illness, may be caused by dependence on others, which undermines self-worth and self-efficacy. Loss of dignity may be associated with hopelessness, a loss of meaning, and a wish for a hastened death.[33]

The Dignity Model, shown in **Table 9**,[34] is a theoretical framework from which to understand the broad issues that impact a person's sense of dignity at the end of life. This model proposes important domains to assess and specific interventions to help patients obtain a sense of dignity. One intervention involves administering a set protocol of questions with themes such as role preservation, pride, hope, and continuity of self.[33] After administering the questions, a transcript is edited into a document with a narrative format that can be reviewed by the patient and shared with loved ones. The purpose of dignity therapy is to provide a sense of meaning and purpose at the end of life. It has been shown to be highly effective. **Table 10** and **Table 11** present another protocol for dignity therapy.

Table 9. The Dignity Model[34]

Major Dignity Categories, Themes, and Subthemes

Illness-Related Concerns	Dignity-Conserving Repertoire	Social-Dignity Inventory
Level of Independence Cognitive acuity Functional capacity **Symptom Distress** Physical distress Psychological distress • medical uncertainty • death anxiety	**Dignity-Conserving Perspectives** Continuity of self Role preservation Generativity/legacy Maintenance of pride Hopefulness Autonomy/control Acceptance Resilience/fighting spirit **Dignity-Conserving Practices** Living "in the moment" Maintaining normalcy Seeking spiritual comfort	Privacy boundaries Social support Care tenor Burden to others Aftermath concerns

Table 10. Dignity Themes, Definitions, and Dignity-Therapy Implications[34,35]

Dignity Theme	Definition	Dignity-Therapy Implication
Generativity	The notion that, for some patients, dignity is intertwined with a sense that one's life has stood for something or has some influence transcendent of death	Sessions are tape-recorded and transcribed, with an edited transcript or "generativity document" being returned to the patient to bequeath to a friend or family member
Continuity of Self	Being able to maintain a feeling that one's essence is intact despite advancing illness	Patients are invited to speak to issues that are foundational to their sense of personhood or self
Role Preservation	Being able to maintain a sense of identification with one or more previously held roles	Patients are questioned about previous or currently held roles that may contribute to their core identity
Maintenance of Pride	An ability to sustain a sense of positive self-regard	Providing opportunities to speak about accomplishments or achievements that engender a sense of pride
Hopefulness	Hopefulness relates to the ability to find or maintain a sense of meaning or purpose	Patients are invited to engage in a therapeutic process intended to instill a sense of meaning and purpose
Aftermath Concerns	Worries or fears concerning the burden or challenges that their death will impose on others	Inviting the patient to speak to issues that might prepare their loved ones for a future without them
Care Tenor	Refers to the attitude and manner with which others interact with the patient that may or may not promote dignity	The tenor of dignity therapy is empathic, nonjudgmental, encouraging, and respectful

From Chochinov HM, Hack T, McClement S, Kristjanson LJ, Harlos M. Dignity therapy: a novel psychotherapeutic intervention for patients near the end of life. J Clin Oncol. 2005;23(24):5520-5525.[33] © 2005 American Society of Clinical Oncology. Reprinted with permission.

Table 11. Dignity Psychotherapy Question Protocol

Tell me a little about your life history; particularly the parts that you either remember most or think are the most important. When did you feel most alive?

Are there specific things that you would want your family to know about you, and are there particular things you would want them to remember?

What are the most important roles you have played in life (family roles, vocational roles, community-service roles, etc.)? Why were they so important to you, and what do you think you accomplished in those roles?

What are your most important accomplishments, and what do you feel most proud of?

Are there particular things that you feel still need to be said to your loved ones or things that you would want to take the time to say once again?

What are your hopes and dreams for your loved ones?

What have you learned about life that you would want to pass along to others? What advice or words of guidance would you wish to pass along to your (son, daughter, husband, wife, parents, other[s])?

Are there words or perhaps even instructions that you would like to offer your family to help prepare them for the future?

In creating this permanent record, are there other things that you would like included?

From Chochinov HM, Hack T, McClement S, Kristjanson LJ, Harlos M. Dignity therapy: a novel psychotherapeutic intervention for patients near the end of life. J Clin Oncol. 2005;23(24):5520-5525.[33] *© 2005 American Society of Clinical Oncology. Reprinted with permission.*

The Universal Need for Meaning

He had but to recall what he had been three months before and what he was now, to recall with what regularity he had been going downhill, for every possibility of hope to be shattered.[36]

—*Tolstoy,* The Death of Ivan Ilych

The need for meaning is universal; meaning provides a sense of purpose and connection in people's lives.[12] Victor Frankl, the founder of logotherapy, and many others have survived extreme loss and privation because they were able to find meaning in the midst of suffering.[37]

Common Sources and Components of Meaning

The most common sources of meaning provide connections with something larger than an individual's own life (eg, family, career, a religious or philosophical system of belief). To be satisfying, a source of meaning must provide a sense of purpose, value, efficacy, and self-worth.

When a particular source of meaning is no longer adequate, people tend to enhance and strengthen their remaining sources of meaning. For example, when terminally ill patients lose the ability to work, they often turn to family or the transcendent realm for a renewed sense of meaning and connection.[12]

Reestablishing a Sense of Meaning

Because the profound losses associated with terminal illness threaten to destroy all sources of meaning, patients and family members may undergo an agonizing search for a renewed sense of meaning as they try to make sense of events and reestablish a sense of wholeness, purpose, and connection. For example, people tend to believe their worth as human beings is defined solely by the following roles:

- independent and energetic member of society
- good provider
- caring parent, son or daughter, spouse, or friend
- productive worker
- discerning intellectual
- healthy athlete
- potent lover.

When profound illness robs people of the energy necessary to sustain their usual roles, the dire meanings they attach to their changed status may cause suffering. For example, on some level, people often believe the following statements:

- Weakness and dependence diminish my worth. Because a terminal illness results in increasing weakness and dependence, my worth will continue to diminish as I become sicker, weaker, and more dependent.
- People love me because of the things I do. As I become sicker, people will cease to love me because the illness will interfere with my ability to perform certain roles.

This suffering can be alleviated by gradually letting go of former roles, but the process is not easy. Usually, terminally ill patients experience prolonged periods of grappling with painful, often unspoken questions, such as the following[32]:

- Who am I now that I can no longer do all the things I used to do?
- Will people still love me and care for me when I smell bad, look bad, and depend on them for everything, including all my personal needs?
- Who am I after I sustain such terrible losses?
- What is happening to me and why is it happening to me?
- How is this going to affect me now and in the future?
- How can I go on in the face of such terrible losses?
- Am I to blame? Did I deserve to have this terrible thing happen to me?
- Am I being punished by God for something I did?
- Will my life ever again contain moments of joy or happiness?
- Will I be abandoned, or will people help me endure and find meaning in my current situation?

As they search for meaning, most patients, family members, and physicians begin to realize they are unlikely to find one common answer to questions such as, "What is the meaning of my life?" "Why is this terrible thing happening?" Instead, they are more likely to find solace by exploring questions of meaning with caring and supportive listeners.

Reconstructing Meaning

Palliative caregivers can alleviate suffering by supporting a patient's efforts to rebuild and reconstruct meaning. Interventions designed to enlarge the patient's sense of purpose, value, efficacy, and self-worth can effectively serve more than one goal. For example,

encouraging patients to tell their life stories gives them a powerful opportunity to reestablish a sense of wholeness and recognize themes of purpose and value in their lives.[11,31,38,39]

Table 12 describes the impact a profound loss is likely to have on four aspects of sources of meaning and offers interventions to reconstruct meaning. The interventions often take less time than some physicians fear and result in a much more rewarding medical practice. When physicians and patients work together to explore the mysteries of meaning and the process of adapting to loss, the result is a strengthened physician-patient relationship, personal healing, and professional satisfaction and growth.

Table 12. Effect of Profound Loss on Four Aspects of Meaning		
Aspect of Meaning	**Effect of Profound Loss**	**Interventions to Reconstruct Meaning**
Purpose		***Develop a Wider Context of Meaning***
Directing activity toward a future or possible state	News of a terminal illness may shift the focus from future goals to an often-disappointing assessment of the actual accomplishments of a lifetime.	Acknowledge the struggle for a sense of purpose, and recognize the impossibility of identifying a single purpose for an entire life.
		Acknowledge the pain of a lost sense of purpose.
		Acknowledge the pain of unfulfilled goals and unrealized dreams and expectations
		Help patients focus on short-term achievable goals.
Extrinsic: goals (short- and long-term)	As death approaches, past achievements and goals that once filled life with a sense of purpose may now seem pointless.	Help patients redirect and enlarge their focus. Encourage patients to reminisce about past sources of joy and fulfillment, identify current sources of satisfaction, and develop concrete short-term plans for engaging in fulfilling activities.
		Encourage patients to review family photograph albums and to tell their life stories.
Intrinsic: fulfillment	Death also signals the end of possibilities; no longer will there be time to realize unfulfilled hopes and dreams.	Help patients explore contexts of meaning that are larger than their individual selves.
		Help patients redirect and enlarge their world view and their sense of self.
		Help patients reframe a situation.

continued

Table 12. Effect of Profound Loss on Four Aspects of Meaning *(continued)*

Aspect of Meaning	Effect of Profound Loss	Interventions to Reconstruct Meaning
Value Feeling that past and current actions are good, justifiable, positive	Patients may examine past behavior and question the value of past actions. Patients may question whether existence will be valued by others. (Will anyone remember me after I die, or will I be completely forgotten?)	***Let Go of Unfinished Business and Accept Forgiveness*** Acknowledge the difficulty of reestablishing a sense of value. Reassure patients that unfinished business is part of the fabric of life. Completing unfinished business could focus on expressing love and asking for and granting forgiveness to self and others. Encourage patients to reconcile their differences with family members, make important final communications, and reaffirm their feelings and wishes. Arrange for appropriate religious rituals and observances, if the patient desires. Encourage patients to explore higher-level meaning for what they have done and are doing. People often generate positive meanings when asked to tell their life stories. Reframe the period of illness and incapacitation by comparing it with the time before illness, if appropriate. This helps patients define their lives in terms broader than just the final illness. Help patients establish a sense of connection with their own definition of ultimate reality, if possible. Shift the patient's focus to less demanding topics when they are too distressed or tired to continue thinking about the meaning of the current situation.
Efficacy Belief in ability to control the self and the environment	Patients may be threatened by loss of control over body, emotions, environment, plans, decision making. Medical settings contribute to sense of vulnerability and helplessness.	***Support Growth and Let Go of Obsessive Need to Control*** Encourage patients to participate in decisions about treatments and family matters. This will help them retain a sense of control. Teach patients and families new coping strategies, such as relaxation, reframing, assertiveness, and effective communication skills. Identify past strengths and successful coping strategies. Ask specific questions to help patients and families develop their own explanations for events. Continue to communicate as much updated information about disease status and treatment options as patients desire. Encourage patients to engage in the ultimate process of letting go, when appropriate.
Self-Worth Need for self-respect and respect from others	Profound illness shatters the assumption that good things happen to good people. Patients often feel as if they are not receiving the good rewards they deserve. Patients may think they are being punished for past misdeeds.	***Reestablish Self-Worth—Enlarge the Sense of Self*** Exhibit interest in patients. Practice active listening with supportive verbal interventions and occasional interpretation. Encourage patients to reminisce and tell their stories. Validate the patient's experiences. Ask questions and make observations about recurring themes. View death as a natural part of the ongoing cycle of life.

Psychological Pain

Losses Associated with Terminal Illness

Most of the time people believe their life seems reasonably predictable and appears to make sense. When a major loss or the threat of a major loss shatters their assumptions about the world, most people feel a painful sense of isolation, brokenness, and sudden loss of meaning.[12]

Terminal illness is associated with major losses. Even a quick reading of the potential losses listed in **Table 13** should help physicians understand the tremendous challenges that dying patients and their families confront as they try to come to terms with approaching death.

Reactions to Loss

Reactions to loss vary widely depending on the nature of the loss, its perceived threats to a person's sense of self, and the person's past experiences, personality, values, and outlook on life. For example, the losses associated with brief periods of illness or the timely and expected death of a distant, elderly relative generally result in temporary distress followed by fairly rapid acceptance of the inevitability of periodic illness and death. Traumatic events such as news of a terminal diagnosis or the unexpected death of a child are likely to cause profoundly disturbing reactions because the associated losses pose tremendous challenges to the individual's sense of self and assumptions about reality.

The reactions described in **Table 14** commonly occur in the face of anticipated or experienced losses; they are part of the grieving process and are not considered pathological unless they become completely disabling or continue unchanged for months or years at a time.

Even normal reactions to loss can be so distressing that patients and family members may think they are abnormal. Clinicians can help normalize common reactions by listening, educating patients and family members about common reactions to loss, reassuring them that such feelings are normal, and encouraging

Table 13. Losses Associated with Terminal Illness
Physical and Intellectual
Short-term memory
Mental, physical, and sexual functioning
Limbs, other body parts, the entire body
Sense of good health and physical well-being
Control over personal environment and bodily functions
Social
Family members
Friends
Political and civic life
Religious community
Emotional and Psychological
Perceived future, hopes, and dreams
Self-image
Secret life
Emotional self-control
Privacy and freedom
Roles in life, such as parent, child, nurturer, chauffeur, breadwinner, cook, lover
Spiritual
Trust in God
Sense of grounding or connection with the transcendent
Sense of wholeness
Sense of purpose, value, worth
Sense of hope and meaning

them to attend support groups in which they can express their feelings.

Adaptation to Loss

Grieving

Many authors previously referenced in this book have explored loss and the search for meaning.[8,12,32] Baumeister, for example, describes an "assumptive world" and suggests that, to maintain a sense of order and control over their existence, people make false assumptions such as the following[12]:

Table 14. Common Reactions to Loss

Physical Sensations

Tightness in chest or throat

Hollowness in the stomach

Oversensitivity to noise

Dry mouth

Breathlessness, feeling short of breath

Weakness in the muscles

Lack of energy

Sense of depersonalization and disconnection

Cognitions

Disbelief

Confusion and difficulty concentrating

Preoccupation with the deceased and obsessive thoughts related to the death

Sense of deceased's presence

Transient thoughts of not wanting to go on living or of not being able to make it through life without the deceased

Dreams about the deceased

Brief visual and auditory hallucinations of the deceased

Denial of the death and associated feelings of grief

Behaviors

Absent-mindedness

Social withdrawal

Sleep disturbances

Restless overactivity

Crying

Appetite disturbances

Sighing

Avoiding reminders of the deceased

Visiting places and carrying objects that remind the survivor of the deceased

Searching and calling out for the deceased

Dreaming about the deceased

Treasuring objects that belonged to the deceased

High levels of fatigue with listlessness and apathy

Disorganization

Feelings

Sadness, frequently accompanied by tears

Shock and numbness

Anger at the deceased for dying, at God for allowing the death, at physicians, etc.

Guilt and self-reproach

Anxiety and depression

Rapid mood changes and irritability

Loneliness and a sense of helplessness

Despair, anguish, and yearning for the deceased

Disconnection from self and others, isolation, and sense of being lost

Disconnection from the transcendent realm, spiritual disorganization, loss of faith and/or religious beliefs

Sense of the world as unreasonable, unpredictable, and dangerous

Sense of being broken, split apart, and disconnected

Loss of purpose and direction

Loss of hope, trust, and meaning

Periodic thoughts of not wanting to go on living

Relief and emancipation

- The world is always a benevolent place.
- As good people, good things will happen to us.
- In general, people get what they deserve.

When traumatic losses occur, these types of assumptions are severely challenged. Suddenly the world becomes a frightening place and the illusion of invulnerability is shattered—good people feel they are not getting what they deserve and bad things are happening to them.[12] In the face of shattered assumptions and lost meaning, it is difficult for patients and family members to continue viewing themselves as powerful, worthwhile, and deserving. Instead, they may be left dangling above an abyss of uncertainty as they desperately try to cope with their losses and make sense of what is happening to them.

However, in the terrible void that causes suffering, both psychological and spiritual healing are possible. In general, adaptation to loss is a process that involves rebuilding an assumptive world by making sense of the loss through reconstructing meaning[12] and opening to an enlarged sense of self associated with the timeless flow of life rather than with previous, limited roles.

As the end of life approaches, patients and family members must adapt to both experienced and anticipated losses. There is a simultaneous and overlapping grief process that occurs both for patients and for family members or caregivers; patients grieve for their ongoing physical and social losses as well as anticipated death, and family members or caregivers grieve for the anticipated death of the patient. Patients must somehow adapt to the approaching loss of everything they have ever known and loved, and family members must learn to cope with losses associated with the patient's increasing incapacity. With enough time and emotional and spiritual support, most terminally ill patients adjust to the inevitability of death, and most family members successfully adapt to loss and eventually move on with their lives.

However, the ability to adapt to loss—or achieve some resolution of grief and go on with life—does not mean the process is short lived or easy. In many cases the process is more protracted and painful than expected. Depending on the nature of the loss, adaptation may involve a matter of weeks or months (eg, when an adult grieves the expected death of a distant, elderly relative), or the process may involve years (eg, when the loss involves the violent or unexpected death of a spouse, child, or sibling). Research has demonstrated a correlation between overwhelming grief and substance abuse. Parents who have lost a child are more likely to experience comorbidities related to substance abuse.[40]

Successfully adapting to loss does not mean the grieving person never experiences loss-related sadness again. As terminally ill patients experience successive losses, grief is likely to resurface with each new loss. For mourners, the first or second anniversaries of the death are frequently associated with acute grief reactions that may last for weeks. Unexpected reminders may trigger renewed episodes of grief for years after the death. However, as adaptation and healing occur, such episodes typically cause less emotional pain and pass more quickly. It is important to remember that most people eventually integrate their losses and go on with their lives.

The Process of Grief

Grief is not an illness that can be cured; it is a normal, multidimensional, unique, dynamic process characterized by pervasive distress to a perceived loss.[41]

Acute grief and its associated bereavement should have a finite period of duration. Recent literature suggests the stage models of grief are inadequate because they fail to address the complexities and variations of the grieving process. See **Figure 1** for a model showing the continuous process of grief such as that seen in older women whose husbands received hospice care.

Tasks of Grief

The tasks of grief and subsequent adjustment to loss involves coping with two main stressors: the loss of a significant person and moving on with life.[42] Worden suggests that people experiencing a significant loss need to complete the four tasks of grief[43]:
- Accept the reality of the loss.
- Experience the pain of the loss.
- Adjust to an environment without the deceased.
- Emotionally relocate the deceased and move on with life.

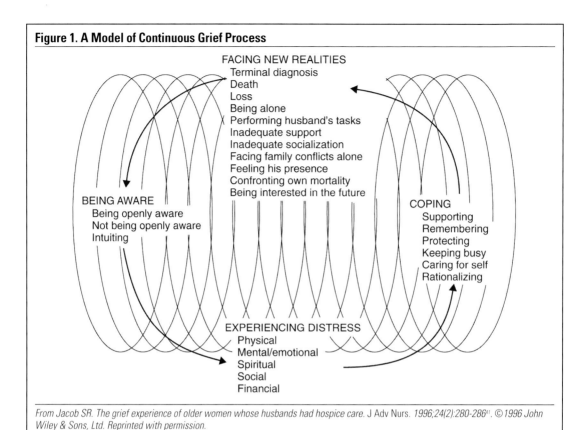

Figure 1. A Model of Continuous Grief Process

FACING NEW REALITIES
Terminal diagnosis
Death
Loss
Being alone
Performing husband's tasks
Inadequate support
Inadequate socialization
Facing family conflicts alone
Feeling his presence
Confronting own mortality
Being interested in the future

BEING AWARE
Being openly aware
Not being openly aware
Intuiting

COPING
Supporting
Remembering
Protecting
Keeping busy
Caring for self
Rationalizing

EXPERIENCING DISTRESS
Physical
Mental/emotional
Spiritual
Social
Financial

From Jacob SR. The grief experience of older women whose husbands had hospice care. J Adv Nurs. 1996;24(2):280-286[41]. ©1996 John Wiley & Sons, Ltd. Reprinted with permission.

After the first task—accepting the reality of the loss—there is no set order for completing the other tasks. Maciewski, on the other hand, demonstrated that the stages of grief do not follow a step-by-step approach. In a study in which caregivers were interviewed during a 24-month period, the grief indicators identified were disbelief, acceptance, yearning, anger, and depression. The most frequent negative response throughout the study period was yearning.[44]

Anxiety and Depression
Characteristic Responses to Disease-Related Stress

Most terminally ill patients are psychologically healthy people who respond to the stresses associated with their illness in a similar pattern.[45] First, there is an initial period of shock and disbelief, followed by a period of turmoil with anxiety and depressive symptoms, irritability, disturbed appetite and sleep, impaired ability to concentrate and perform the usual tasks of daily living, and intrusive thoughts about the illness and fears of the future. Then patients begin to the process of adaptation. In many cases, as the adaptive response occurs, emotional distress resolves, particularly when patients receive support from family members, friends, and physicians. During the adaptive period, appropriate interventions include the caring presence and supportive interventions offered by all members of the interdisciplinary team, including physicians, nurses, social workers, and chaplains; effective control of physical symptoms and encouragement to exercise and eat well, if possible; and a short course of insomnia medication.[45]

Prevalence of Anxiety and Depression

Although more than half of patients adjust to the periodic episodes of profound emotional distress that commonly occur during the course of any terminal illness, the remaining patients experience clinically apparent psychiatric disorders, the most common of which are reactive anxiety and depression and major depression.[14]

Persistent, high levels of anxiety and depression are not adaptive; they require aggressive intervention, including short-term psychotherapy and anxiolytic and antidepressant drugs.[40] Skilled intervention is needed whenever anxiety or depression worsens, interferes with the patient's ability to function, or persists for more than 7 days.[46]

Anxiety and depression are the most common forms of psychological distress for terminally ill patients.[47] However, the prevalence of anxiety and depression varies considerably depending on the type of disease,[48] the stage and site of disease, the patient's coping ability, and the amount of emotional support from family and friends.[49]

In one study of the prevalence of psychiatric disorders among cancer patients, 47% met criteria for a psychiatric disorder.[50] Of the 47%, more than two-thirds had reactive anxiety or depression (adjustment disorders with depressed or anxious mood), 13% had major depression, and 8% had an organic mental disorder (delirium). At Memorial Sloan-Kettering Cancer Center, more than half of the patients referred to the psychiatric service for evaluation were diagnosed as having adjustment disorders, usually with features of anxiety and depression.[51]

In another study of 62 oncology patients, approximately 24% experienced severe depressive symptoms; the prevalence increased to 77% among those with advanced illness.[14,52]

Short-Term Psychotherapy

When short-term psychotherapy is initiated to help relieve anxiety and depression, family members should be included when appropriate, and emphasis should be placed on the following[14,46]:

- Provide as much updated information about treatment and prognosis as the patient desires.
- Correct misconceptions about the past and present with honest and compassionate communication.
- Educate patients and family members about the

psychological, biological, and pharmacological factors that contribute to anxiety and depression.
- Integrate the terminal illness into the patient's entire life experience.
- Establish attainable, short-term goals and expectations.
- Identify and emphasize the patient's past strengths and successful coping techniques, including distraction, short-term psychotherapy, journaling, and exercise.
- Teach relaxation techniques, such as focusing on passive breathing (the natural rhythms of breathing), accompanied by either passive or active muscle relaxation, meditation, guided imagery, or self-hypnosis to help reduce anxiety and increase the patient's sense of control.
- Provide ongoing emotional support and caring presence to reduce the patient's sense of isolation.
- Help the patient reestablish a sense of self-worth.

Drug Therapy Guidelines

In most cases, the pharmacological management of anxiety and depression is fairly straightforward. The more complicated task, which can test the skills of the most experienced clinician, is distinguishing the normal sadness and anxiety associated with dying from major depression and anxiety, which require pharmacological treatment and/or short-term psychotherapy. When medication is needed to control anxiety and depression, it is important to select drugs with the fewest negative side effects and to use the lowest possible dosages consistent with effective symptom relief.

Assessing and Managing Anxiety

Periodic anxiety is a normal and expected consequence of the uncertainties of illness and approaching death; however, high levels of persistent anxiety are not an inevitable part of the dying process.[14] In hospice and palliative care settings anxiety is generally described as a feeling of helplessness or fear, often generated by death-related factors. **Table 15** describes events associated with periods of increased anxiety. When assessing for anxiety, a careful history and physical examination are the most important first steps for providing effective interventions. Initial emphasis should be placed on

Table 15. Periodic Anxiety: Associated Events and Overall Content
Events Associated with Periods of Increased Anxiety
Initial diagnosis
Occurrence of persistent symptoms
Recurrence or progression of disease
Changes in treatment
Anniversary of illness-related events
Terminal stage of illness
Content of Anxiety
Fear of uncontrolled pain (or other uncontrolled symptoms)
Fear of isolation or abandonment
Fear of loss of control
Fear of inability to cope
Fear of becoming a burden

identifying treatable medical complications (eg, pain, anxiety caused by medications), but physicians should try to rule out other common contributing factors, such as psychological, social, and spiritual pain.[53]

Patients with dyspnea tend to be the most anxious; however, remarkable relief can usually be obtained with opioid therapy.[54] (See UNIPAC 4.)

When managing anxiety, the following factors should be considered:

- the patient's subjective level of distress and symptom severity
- problematic patient behavior and functional impairment
- the duration of anxiety (ie, longer than 1 or 2 weeks)
- the family's reaction to the patient's distress and their coping resources
- treatable causes that may improve (eg, physical, psychosocial, spiritual)
- benefits versus burdens of potential treatments
- the resources of the entire team
- the patient's responses to caring human contact, education, supportive counseling, and short-term psychotherapy and interventions designed to enhance purpose, value, efficacy, and self-worth.

See **Table 16** for the diagnostic criteria for generalized anxiety disorder from the DSM-IV-TR.[55] See **Table 17** for causes, symptoms, and remedies for anxiety.

Table 16. Diagnostic Criteria for Generalized Anxiety Disorder

A. Excessive anxiety and worry (apprehensive expectation), occurring more days than not for at least 6 months, about a number of events or activities (such as work or school performance).

B. The person finds it difficult to control the worry.

C. The anxiety and worry are associated with 3 (or more) of the following 6 symptoms (with at least some symptoms present for more days than not for the past 6 months). Note: Only 1 item is required in children.
    (1) restlessness or feeling keyed up or on edge
    (2) being easily fatigued
    (3) difficulty concentrating or mind going blank
    (4) irritability
    (5) muscle tension
    (6) sleep disturbance (difficulty falling or staying asleep, or restless unsatisfying sleep).

D. The focus of the anxiety and worry is not confined to features of an Axis I disorder; the anxiety or worry is not about having a panic attack (as in panic disorder), being embarrassed in public (as in social phobia), being contaminated (as in obsessive-compulsive disorder), being away from home or close relatives (as in separation anxiety disorder), gaining weight (as in anorexia nervosa), having multiple physical complaints (as in somatization disorder), or having a serious illness (as in hypochondriasis), and the anxiety and worry do not occur exclusively during posttraumatic stress disorder.

E. The anxiety, worry, or physical symptoms cause clinically significant distress or impairment in social, occupational, or other important areas of functioning.

F. The disturbance is not due to the direct physiological effects of a substance (eg, a drug of abuse, a medication) or a general medical condition (eg, hyperthyroidism) and does not occur exclusively during a mood disorder, a psychotic disorder, or a pervasive developmental disorder.

Summarized from the Diagnostic and Statistical Manual of Mental Disorders Text Revision, *4th edition, by the American Psychiatric Association.*[55]

Table 17. Anxiety: Causes, Symptoms, and Remedies[56]

Causes

Situational

Worry about family, finances

Fear of the unknown, hospital, treatment

Isolation, inadequate support

Role loss, sense of uselessness

Uncertainty, lack of information, misinformation

Caused by Drugs

Corticosteroids

Drug-induced hallucinations

Benzodiazepines or opioids

Withdrawal states precipitated by abrupt discontinuation of benzodiazepines, alcohol, opioids

Organic

Uncontrolled pain and other symptoms

Dyspnea, hypoxia, increasing respiratory effort

Weakness

Hypoglycemia, sepsis, fever, hypertension

Insomnia

Brain tumor

Adverse drug reactions such as akathisia or myoclonus

Psychological

Denial, anger, guilt, fear

Preexisting anxiety disorders (eg, exaggerated reaction)

Preexisting anxiety disorders (panic disorders, obsessive-compulsive disorder, phobias)

Depression

Delirium

Causes Related to Patient's Inner World

Existential distress, hopelessness, meaninglessness

Fear of mental impairment

Fear of loss of independence

Fear of pain

Thoughts about death

Thoughts about the past (eg, wasted opportunities, guilt)

Look For

Persistent tenseness

Inability to relax

Worry, fearfulness, dread

More than normal mood variation

Poor concentration

Impaired ability to assimilate or recall information

Rumination, intrusive thoughts

Indecisiveness

Insomnia

Irritability, restlessness

Inability to distract self or be distracted

Panic attacks

Sweating, tremors

Nausea, anorexia

Shortness of breath, hyperventilation

Consider

Nonpharmacological

- Multidisciplinary assessments
- Treatment of reversible causes
- Short-term psychotherapy

If the above are ineffective, consider pharmacological interventions

Pharmacological

Simple anxiety: benzodiazepines such as

Short-acting

- lorazepam, 0.5 to 2 mg PO two to four times daily. Peaks in 1 to 6 hours. Liquid available. Other routes: SL, PR, IV.
- alprazolam, 0.25 to 2 mg PO or SL three to four times daily (max. 10 mg/24 hours). Peaks in 30 minutes. Other routes: SL, PR. Short halflife; quick relief of acute anxiety.

Long-acting

- diazepam, 2 to 20 mg PO every day, three times daily. Peaks in 15 to 45 minutes. Liquid formulation available. Other routes: SL, PR, IV. Long half-life; steady plasma concentration.
- clonazepam, 0.25 to 0.5 PO two to three times daily up to 4 mg per day.

Severe anxiety or anxiety with paranoia, hallucinations: major tranquilizers such as

- haloperidol, 0.5 to 4 mg twice daily and every 4 hours, as needed. Peaks in 3 to 6 hours. Liquid available. Other routes: SL, PR, SC, IV.

If the above are ineffective or if the patient is unable to take oral medications, consider

- midazolam, 1 mg SC/IV stat or titrated to relief by SC infusion.

Assessing and Managing Depression

Differentiating expected emotional distress associated with a terminal illness (sadness, grief, and bereavement) from the psychiatric disorder of major depression presents challenges for many clinicians.[57-59]

During the course of a terminal illness, many patients experience periodic, brief episodes of intense sadness accompanied by depressive symptoms such as crying. During the spiritual process of letting go, some patients experience a sense of despair. In these situations, patients are unlikely to benefit from pharmacological treatment. Instead, they need caring support as they search for meaning and adapt to changing roles. (For more information, see the chapter "Spiritual Pain" on page 55.)

Depression is common in terminally ill patients and their family caregivers; a significant percentage develops reactive and major depression during the course of a terminal illness.[60] A study by van der Lee and colleagues revealed that 15% to 25% of terminally ill cancer patients also have depression.[61]

Depression is associated with inappropriate and excessive guilt, thoughts of death, prolonged functional impairment, hallucinations (other than transitory auditory or visual hallucinations of the deceased, common during bereavement)[55], and persistent, overwhelming feelings of despair, hopelessness, and worthlessness. Depression is a source of intense emotional pain, and its vigorous treatment is mandated by the goals of hospice and palliative medicine. Depression is not a necessary, normal, or required part of the dying process. Despite the fact that oncologists feel competent managing depression, only 55% reported being effective at identifying and diagnosing depression.[62]

Common Causes of Depressive Symptoms

Because depressive symptoms have multiple causes (eg, exhaustion, uncontrolled pain, medication, fear of being a burden to others, loss of purpose and meaning, religious concerns), a thorough history and physical examination are essential first steps to providing effective interventions. During the assessment process, initial emphasis should be placed on identifying treatable medical causes of depressive symptoms. **Table 18** describes the diagnosis of major depressive disorder, summarized from the DSM-IV-TR.

Risk Factors for Depression

The following factors increase a patient's risk of developing depression[46]:

- poorly controlled pain
- family history of depression
- history of affective disorder or alcoholism
- advanced stage of illness
- increased physical impairment
- left hemispheric strokes[48]
- pancreatic cancer
- other illnesses such as hypothyroidism often associated with depressive symptoms
- treatment with certain medications such as clonidine or propranolol.

Assessment and Measurement Tools

Most cases of depression are undetected by physicians and other healthcare providers unless they systematically use a screening instrument for depression.[53] Simple, straightforward questions often result in important information from the patient. In most cases, patients welcome the opportunity to discuss their concerns and feelings. When depression is suspected, practitioners should sit near the patient and gently ask simple questions such as the following[18]:

- How has your mood been recently?
- Have you been tearful lately?
- Can you tell me more about how you're feeling?
- Do you think you might be depressed?
- Have you ever been depressed? Did you get treatment? Was the treatment effective?

A validated one-question screening item is, "Are you depressed?" This has been compared to a two-item screen, the Beck Depression Inventory-Short Form, and a visual analog scale and found to be superior in sensitivity and specificity to diagnose minor and major depression in the terminally ill.[63]

Short, easy-to-use assessment scales that focus on psychological and cognitive symptoms and suicidal ideation can reliably determine the presence of depression in dying patients. See **Table 19** for the Center for Epidemiologic Studies-Depression (CES-D) Boston Short Form.

The 10-item version of the CES-D (sometimes referred to as the Boston Short Form) is the briefest and

Table 18. Diagnosis of Major Depressive Disorder, Single Episode

A. The person experiences a single major depressive episode:
1. For a major depressive episode, a person must have experienced at least five of the nine symptoms below for the same 2 weeks or more, for most of the time almost every day, and this is a change from his/her prior level of functioning. One of the symptoms must be either (a) depressed mood, or (b) loss of interest.
   a. Depressed mood. For children and adolescents, this may be irritable mood.
   b. A significantly reduced level of interest or pleasure in most or all activities.
   c. A considerable loss or gain of weight (eg, 5% or more change of weight in a month when not dieting). This may also be an increase or decrease in appetite. For children, they may not gain an expected amount of weight.
   d. Difficulty falling or staying asleep (insomnia), or sleeping more than usual (hypersomnia).
   e. Behavior that is agitated or slowed down. Others should be able to observe this.
   f. Feeling fatigued, or diminished energy.
   g. Thoughts of worthlessness or extreme guilt (not about being ill).
   h. Ability to think, concentrate, or make decisions is reduced.
   i. Frequent thoughts of death or suicide (with or without a specific plan), or attempt of suicide.
2. The person's symptoms do not indicate a mixed episode.
3. The person's symptoms are a cause of great distress or difficulty in functioning at home, work, or other important areas.
4. The person's symptoms are not caused by substance use (eg, alcohol, drugs, medication) or a medical disorder.
5. The person's symptoms are not due to normal grief or bereavement over the death of a loved one, they continue for more than 2 months, or they include great difficulty in functioning, frequent thoughts of worthlessness, thoughts of suicide, symptoms that are psychotic, or behavior that is slowed down (psychomotor retardation).

B. Another disorder does not better explain the major depressive episode.

C. The person has never had a manic, mixed, or a hypomanic episode (unless an episode was due to a medical disorder or use of a substance).

Summarized from the Diagnostic and Statistical Manual of Mental Disorders Text Revision, *4th edition, by the American Psychiatric Association.*[55]

Table 19. Screening for Depression with CES-D Boston Short Form

Ask: Did you experience the following much of the time during the past week?

Yes	No	Item
X		I felt depressed.
X		I felt that everything I did was an effort.
X		My sleep was restless.
	X	I was happy.
X		I felt lonely.
X		People were unfriendly.
	X	I enjoyed life.
X		I felt sad.
X		I felt that people disliked me.
X		I could not get going.

Scoring: The user sums the scores of all items by counting the responses to the items above. Items in which a person with depression is likely to answer "no," such as "I was happy" and "I enjoyed life" are scored in reverse (ie, "no" responses add points to depression score).

simplest version available of the widely used and validated CES-D scale.[64-66] The CES-D detects depression in patients and caregivers and monitors mood changes over time. Research indicates that people scoring 4 or higher on the instrument have a high probability of depression, whereas individuals scoring 3 or lower have a low probability. The instrument should not be used by itself to diagnose depression; additional questions must be asked to diagnose specific depressive disorders and plan treatment. Repeated administration of the instrument over time provides valuable information, both for clinical purposes and program development.

A useful screening tool for depression in the elderly is the Geriatric Depression Scale (Short Form), a 15-item questionnaire that can be completed in less than 5 minutes, shown in **Table 20.**

Causes, Symptoms, and Pharmacological Treatments

See **Table 21** for common causes and symptoms of depression. Treatment for depression will often involve a combination of pharmacologic and nonpharmacologic therapies such as multidisciplinary assessments and behavioral therapy. Pharmacologic treatments are typically divided into three major categories: selective serotonin reuptake inhibitors (SSRIs), psychostimulants, and tricyclic antidepressants (TCAs). **Table 22** suggests pharmacological treatments for treating major depression.

Selective Serotonin Reuptake Inhibitors

SSRIs are often less sedating and have fewer autonomic side effects. Typical side effects include gastrointestinal upset, sexual dysfunction, tremor, and increased sweating. SSRIs such as fluoxetine are typically more energizing than sertraline and paroxetine. Paroxetine is also associated with increased dry mouth and sweating. Newer

---

Table 20. Geriatric Depression Scale (Short Form)[67,68]

Choose the best answer for how you have felt over the past week:

1.	Are you basically satisfied with your life?	YES/**NO**
2.	Have you dropped many of your activities and interests?	**YES**/NO
3.	Do you feel that your life is empty?	**YES**/NO
4.	Do you often get bored?	**YES**/NO
5.	Are you in good spirits most of the time?	YES/**NO**
6.	Are you afraid something bad is going to happen to you?	**YES**/NO
7.	Do you feel happy most of the time?	YES/**NO**
8.	Do you often feel helpless?	**YES**/NO
9.	Do you prefer to stay at home, rather than going out and doing new things?	**YES**/NO
10.	Do you feel you have more problems with memory than most?	**YES**/NO
11.	Do you think it is wonderful to be alive now?	YES/**NO**
12.	Do you feel pretty worthless the way you are now?	**YES**/NO
13.	Do you feel full of energy?	YES/**NO**
14.	Do you feel that your situation is hopeless?	**YES**/NO
15.	Do you think that most people are better off than you are?	**YES**/NO

Answers in **bold** indicate depression. Although differing sensitivities and specificities have been obtained across studies, for clinical purposes a score > 5 points is suggestive of depression and should warrant a follow-up interview. Scores > 10 are almost always depression.

Note. The Geriatric Depression Rating Scale is available online at the Stanford/VA/NIA Aging Clinical Research Center Web site. Available at: www.stanford.edu/~yesavage/Testing.htm. Accessed March 17, 2008.

Table 21. Depression: Causes and Symptoms

Causes	Look For
Psychiatric Causes	**Psychological Indicators**
• Major depression	• Profound feelings of worthlessness
• Adjustment disorders	• Profound or excessive feelings of guilt
Medical Causes	• Profound anhedonia
• Poorly controlled pain or other physical symptoms	• Profound thoughts of wishing for death
• Drugs (eg, opioids, corticosteroids, diazepam)	• Profound feelings of hopelessness and helplessness
• Tumor involvement of central nervous system	• Suicidal ideation
• Infections (eg, Epstein-Barr virus)	**Somatic Signs and Symptoms**
• Metabolic disturbances (eg, abnormal levels of sodium or calcium)	Less valuable when assessing depression in terminally ill patients; the illness itself can produce symptoms of fatigue, loss of energy, anorexia, and insomnia
• Nutritional problems (eg, anemia or deficiencies in vitamin B12 or folate)	
• Endocrine disorders (eg, hypothyroidism or adrenal insufficiency)	
• Neurological disorders (eg, Parkinson's disease)	
Psychological, Social, and Spiritual Causes	
• Grief	
• Existential distress	
• Concerns about family distress	
• Overwhelming financial or family distress	
• Hopelessness and meaninglessness	
• Guilt	
• Fear of expressing anger	
• Sleep deprivation	

antidepressants including citalopram and escitalopram are typically less sedating. Patients starting SSRIs will often experience temporary nausea and anxiety.

Tricyclic Antidepressants

TCAs are effective for controlling neuropathic pain. Amitriptyline and doxepin are typically more sedating than desipramine or nortriptyline. These medications are associated with various side effects and should be adjusted when negative side effects occur. The therapeutic range is wide, and drug levels can be monitored for most TCAs.

Psychostimulants

Psychostimulants include methylphenidate, dextroamphetamine, and modafinil. These medications have immediate effectiveness and can counter the effects of opioid-induced sedation. The use of psychostimulants can result in the development of anxiety, insomnia, paranoia, psychosis, and tolerance. They should not be administered to patients with severe anxiety disorder, tachyarrhythmia, or angina.

The results of traditional pharmacological therapy may begin to appear within 7 to 10 days, although full benefit may not occur for 2 to 4 weeks. Psychostimulants take effect more quickly. Psychostimulants are useful antidepressant agents when prescribed selectively for terminally ill patients with depression. In addition to their antidepressant properties, they lessen sedation secondary to opioid therapy and are potent adjuvant analgesics. At relatively low dosages, psychostimulants improve appetite, promote a sense of well-being, and reduce feelings of weakness and fatigue. Treatment usually begins with a low dosage that is slowly increased over several days until the desired effect is achieved or until side effects such as agitation, insomnia, and anxiety occur. After a few days, a tricyclic antidepressant can be added to prolong and potentiate the effect of the stimulant.[69] If increased anxiety

Table 22. Examples of Pharmacological Agents for Treating Major Depression in Patients with Advanced Disease

Drug	Dosage	Notes
Selective Seratonin Reuptake Inhibitors: Less sedation and dry mouth than tricyclics; less likely to alleviate neuropathic pain; often reduce libido.		
Citalopram	10 to 20 mg daily ↑ up to 60 mg daily	• Fewer drug interactions • Taper off when discontinuing
Paroxetine	10 mg each am ↑ up to 50 mg every 24 hours	
Sertraline	50 mg each am ↑ up to 200 mg every 24 hours	• For frail elderly, begin with half the usual starting dose.
Escitalopram	10 to 20 mg daily	• Also helpful for treating generalized anxiety disorder. • Well tolerated in the elderly.
Tricyclic Antidepressants: Best-studied; give single dose usually at bedtime. Helpful for insomnia and neuropathic pain. Anticholinergic side effects.		
Amitriptyline	10 to 75 mg PO at bedtime ↑ up to 150 mg every 24 hours	• Sedating, analgesic effects are well studied
Desipramine	10 to 75 mg PO at bedtime ↑ up to 150 mg every 24 hours	• Fewer side effects than amitriptyline, less sedating
Nortriptyline	10 to 25 mg PO at bedtime ↑ up to 75 mg over 3 to 5 days	• Oral solution available, fewer side effects than amitriptyline
Doxepin	10 to 50 mg PO at bedtime ↑ up to 300 mg every 24 hours	• Sedating, fewer side effects than amitriptyline
Miscellaneous Antidepressants: Can be very useful for some patients with anxiety or low energy levels.		
Bupropion	100 mg PO twice daily ↑ up to 300 to 450 mg/day	• Weak serotonin, norepinephrine, and dopamine reuptake inhibitor; useful for low energy; contraindicated with seizures, bulimia, anorexia
Mirtazepine	15 mg at bedtime and ↑ up to 45 mg/day	• Norepinephrine and serotonin antagonist. Possible sedation, weight gain
Venlafaxine	75 mg/day divided doses ↑ up to 375 mg/day	• Useful for some neuropathic pains
Duloxetine	30 to 60 mg/day	• Also indicated for diabetic neuropathic pain
Psychostimulants: Rapid effect, but may exacerbate anxiety and restlessness; taper off slowly if possible.		
Methylphenidate or Dextroamphetamine	2.5 mg at 8 am and noon ↑ gradually to 60 mg every 24 hours	• Doses greater than 30 mg/day are not usually necessary; occasionally, patients require up to 60 mg/day.
Pemoline	18.75 mg at 8 am and noon ↑ gradually up to 75 mg/day	• Patients typically require no more than 75 mg/day. Pemoline comes in chewable tablets that can be absorbed through the buccal mucosa. It should be used with caution in patients with liver impairment.
Benzodiazepines: Helpful when anxiety coexists with depression.		
Alprazolam	0.25 to 1.0 mg three times daily	• Taper off slowly if possible.

or restlessness becomes problematic, taper the stimulant dosage until it can be withdrawn. If no improvement is seen and doubt about the diagnosis exits, a psychiatric consultation should be considered. Most antidepressants can be discontinued without difficulty; however, psychostimulants may need to be discontinued more slowly.

Pharmacological Treatment for Depression in the Elderly and Frail

Treatment of depression in frail and elderly patients requires careful prescribing and close monitoring. Choose an antidepressant with a desired side effect profile; for instance, the sedating effects of antidepressants such as nortriptyline are desired when treating patients with agitated depression and difficulty sleeping.

Use the smallest possible effective dosage of medication to avoid undesired side effects; terminally ill patients may be able to tolerate only a fraction of the usual maximal maintenance antidepressant dosage. SSRIs have fewer sedative and anticholinergic side effects.

Avoid monoamine oxidase inhibitors because of the likelihood of adverse interactions with food and other medications except for patients who have used them previously with good results. Psychostimulants can also be helpful for treating the frail and elderly. See above for more information.

CLINICAL SITUATION

Lewis and Mabel

Lewis, a 62-year-old man, has developed advanced chronic obstructive pulmonary disease after a 30-year history of heavy smoking. During the past 5 years, Lewis has become increasingly debilitated and has required oxygen for the last 2 years. Lewis has been hospitalized three times during the past 3 months; before the most recent admission he was so short of breath he didn't think he was going to live through the night.

Despite maximal treatment with bronchodilators and the addition of high-dose steroids, Lewis's condition remains unimproved. When he refuses another round of intubation and mechanical ventilation in the ICU, the palliative care consultation service introduces the philosophy of hospice care. The team's nurse and social worker describe hospice services and the palliative medicine consultant explains how future episodes of dyspnea might be managed. Lewis says he is ready for anything that will get him out of the hospital. Lewis's wife, Mabel, sits in the corner weeping, but Lewis's grown daughter asks many questions and the family eventually agrees to hospice care.

Lewis is transferred to his home in an ambulance. When the hospice physician and social worker arrive, they find that a particularly rough ambulance ride has left Lewis in a very frightened state. He pleads, "Do something to help me—I can't breathe!"

Question One

At this point, which is the most appropriate action?

A. Complete a rapid but thorough history and physical examination.
B. Send Lewis back to the hospital immediately.
C. Ask if Lewis in interested in an injection of sedatives.
D. Order lorazepam, 1 mg PO, now.

Correct Response and Analysis

A is the correct response. Even a quick history and physical examination are likely to suggest treatments that will relieve Lewis's symptoms and give him and his family enough time to resolve end-of-life issues. B and C are incorrect because they are unnecessary. D is incorrect because lorazepam may not be the most helpful agent to relieve Lewis's symptoms.

The Case Continues

During the course of a focused history and physical examination, it becomes clear that Lewis has advanced emphysema and is very frightened by his symptoms. Ever since Lewis's older brother died of lung cancer while experiencing severe anxiety and shortness of breath, Lewis has been haunted by the memory of his brother's miserable death and is terrified about having to endure a similar fate.

Lewis is too weak to go to the bathroom by himself and is very unhappy about needing so much assistance from Mabel and his daughter. He says he wishes he was already dead. Lewis's medications are theophylline, 300 mg twice a day; albuterol inhaler, two puffs every 4 hours; ipratropium inhaler, two puffs every 4 hours; and prednisone, 20 mg PO every morning.

The physical examination reveals a very anxious, unhappy man with a 35% oxygen mask that makes communication difficult. Lewis is extremely tremulous and complains of sleeplessness at night. He is breathing 35 times a minute, his blood pressure is 150/100, his pulse is 120 beats per minute, his chest is barrel-shaped with very few breath sounds and no rales or wheezes in any lung field, his heart tones are not audible, his abdomen is somewhat distended, he has not had a bowel movement for 8 days, and his feet have 3+ edema.

While Lewis is being examined Mabel sits in the kitchen with the social worker. Mabel tearfully explains that her relationship with Lewis was very strained before his last hospitalization and says that, in the past, Lewis has coped with difficulties by denying their existence, drinking, and watching television. Mabel is afraid that Lewis might commit suicide.

Question Two

At this point, what is the best intervention?
A. Prescribe an antidepressant.
B. Initiate around-the-clock suicide prevention interventions.
C. Treat Lewis's physical symptoms.
D. Teach Lewis how to meditate so he can relax.

Correct Response and Analysis

A is incorrect because it is unlikely to be helpful. If treatable symptoms such as shortness of breath, pain, and constipation are contributing to Lewis's anxiety and depression, providing effective treatments will not only relieve the distressing physical symptoms, but they also may relieve his anxiety and depression and increase his trust in the physician.

B is also incorrect. Suicide interventions are unlikely to be necessary because Lewis is too weak to get out of bed by himself (but the family should make sure he does not have access to toxic pills or guns).

C is the correct response. Because medical complications are likely causes of anxiety and depression in terminally ill patients, treating distressing physical symptoms is the most important first step.

D is incorrect. At this time, attempts to teach meditation are unlikely to be helpful because Lewis's distressing symptoms will interfere with his ability to concentrate on anything else.

The Case Continues

The hospice physician suspects that Lewis is experiencing an agitated depression, exacerbated by shortness of breath, constipation, and family stress. However, before prescribing an antidepressant, the physician focuses on relieving Lewis's physical symptoms and orders the following:

- Double the prednisone dosage to 40 mg per day.
- Continue the albuterol and ipratropium nebulizer every 4 to 6 hours.
- Reduce the theophylline dosage to 150 mg twice a day to relieve tremulousness.
- Add hydrocodone syrup, 3 mg every 4 hours, to help relieve shortness of breath.
- Recommend a potent dose of milk of magnesia or polyethylene glycol and senna tablets to treat and prevent constipation.
- Order physical and respiratory therapy to help Lewis clear his secretions and increase his mobility by teaching him to conserve his energy and transfer from bed to wheelchair.

The hospice physician is able to calm Lewis with careful explanations of what will be done to help him, and Lewis agrees to try the new regimen.

The next day Lewis is a little better and the hydrocodone dose has to be increased to 5 mg every 4 hours. When the hospice nurse visits the following day, Lewis's physical symptoms are much improved. He is sitting in an easy chair and is able to talk. Lewis reports his appetite and shortness of breath have improved, and he feels calmer and less tremulous. Because Lewis can now transfer from bed to wheelchair, the nurse suggests an order for portable oxygen so Lewis can leave the house, but he responds, "What's the use? I might as well be dead." On further questioning, Lewis denies thoughts of suicide, but says he just doesn't feel good and is unable to sleep at night.

Over the next 2 days Lewis's dyspnea seems controlled and a reservoir nasal cannula is substituted for the oxygen mask, but his depressive symptoms worsen. He stops taking his medication, which exacerbates his physical symptoms. Exhausted and frantic, Lewis's daughter calls the hospice program and Lewis is admitted to the hospice inpatient unit for further evaluation and symptom management.

The physician first tries to determine whether Lewis's renewed medical problems are causing his depressive symptoms. Lewis is extremely short of breath and, when questioned, he shakes his head and stares at the floor. The physician turns to Mabel and Lewis's daughter for more information and they report that Lewis has refused his medications for 2 days, appears increasingly despondent, is unwilling to meet with old friends, and does not even watch sports on television, which has always been a big part of his life.

When Lewis's brother is mentioned, Lewis moans and shakes his head adamantly. The physician talks with Lewis about taking his medicine and using his nebulizers again, and, with some encouragement from his family, Lewis agrees to give it one more try. The physician restarts the bronchodilators and steroids and switches the opioid to oxycodone, 5 mg every 4 hours, which may relieve Lewis's increased shortness of breath and allow him to sleep at night.

The next day the physician meets with the team to discuss Lewis's case. The social worker reports the prominent depressive features she noted while Lewis was at home, which included social withdrawal and frequent comments about wishing he were dead. After talking with Lewis's family, the social worker has concluded that Lewis has never had good coping skills; he does not discuss his feelings with anyone and he copes with adversity by drinking beer and watching television. Now that Lewis is less able to use these coping strategies, fearful thoughts about his coming death are likely to be intruding.

The physician suggests a trial of antidepressants and the team concurs, particularly when the social worker mentions that attempts to persuade Lewis to discuss his feelings have so far been unproductive. The physician also recommends more intensive involvement by all members of the team. Later that day the physician visits Lewis, who is feeling somewhat less breathless on the increased opioid dosage (oxycodone, 5 mg every 4 hours). When the physician recommends an antidepressant, Lewis agrees to take any kind of pill but says he is sure it will not help him.

Question Three

At this point, which of the following are appropriate interventions? (Select all that apply.)

A. Decrease the oxycodone to 2 mg every 4 hours and order nortriptyline, 25 mg at bedtime.
B. Increase the oxycodone to 7 mg every 4 hours during the day and 10 mg at night, and order escitalopram, 10 mg a day.
C. Ask the social worker to arrange a family conference with Lewis, his wife, and his daughter.
D. Ask the chaplain to visit with Lewis.

Correct Response and Analysis

B is a better response than A. Increasing the daytime oxycodone dosage is likely to further relieve Lewis's sense of breathlessness and the increased nighttime dosage will probably help him sleep. Although a somewhat sedating tricyclic such as nortriptyline can be an appropriate order for a patient with depression who is also having difficulty sleeping, in this case a less sedating SSRI such as escitalopram is the more appropriate order. A sedating antidepressant may interfere with Lewis's ability to tolerate the increased opioid dosages that he is likely to need as his breathlessness increases.

C is also correct because a skillfully facilitated family conference can help family members discuss issues that have not been addressed. D may also be correct because Lewis may be experiencing spiritual pain.

The Case Concludes

While Lewis is in the inpatient unit, the family has an opportunity to rest, which helps reduce their level of stress. During an initial visit the chaplain discovers that Lewis has rarely attended church but expresses belief in a higher power of some sort and seems to feel guilty about not being more helpful when his brother was dying. Over the next few days the relationship between the chaplain and Lewis improves, particularly when Lewis discovers the chaplain also enjoys sports. Lewis is able to further express the guilt he feels for not having been able to reduce his brother's suffering and talks about his own fears of dying.

During a family conference facilitated by a social worker, Lewis is able to voice his affection for his family, and his wife and daughter are able to voice their love for him and their appreciation for his role as a husband and father. Lewis's daughter is particularly articulate about her affection for her father. As Lewis's depression improves, he is more willing to work with a physical therapist, who compliments him on his progress and shows him techniques to increase his mobility. Lewis requests a discharge saying, "I have things I need to do."

During the course of the next 6 weeks, Lewis's opioid dosage is titrated upward as needed to relieve his increasing sense of breathlessness, and he is reassured that symptom control will continue to receive highest priority. Lewis's talk about suicide does not recur, and he visits briefly with old friends. Members of the hospice home care team, including the chaplain, visit frequently and help provide emotional and spiritual support. On two occasions, when Lewis seems despondent, Mabel asks the chaplain to make extra visits. On each occasion, Lewis reviews his life as a pipe fitter, a husband, and a father and reexamines his role during his brother's death.

The chaplain helps Lewis recognize themes of endurance, hard work, and caring in his life story and encourages Lewis to acknowledge, and then let go of, the guilt he continues to feel for being so helpless during his brother's death. The chaplain also encourages Lewis and Mabel to look at family photographs and reminisce about difficult and happy times during their life together.

When Lewis becomes so weak that he cannot swallow tablets, a subcutaneous infusion of morphine and midazolam is started at home and is titrated upward as needed. The hospice physician visits Lewis at home to provide emotional support and to reassure him that medications will be used to prevent the symptoms Lewis so greatly fears. Lewis dies comfortably in his home with Mabel, his daughter, and the hospice nurse at his bedside.

Treating Refractory Symptoms

On occasion, despite the best efforts of skilled physicians, a small percentage of terminally ill patients continues to endure unrelieved physical, psychological, social, and spiritual pain. In such cases, all members of an interdisciplinary team should be involved in the patient's care and every effort should be made to reassess the patient for contributing factors and possible treatments.

In addition to increased team involvement, consultation with the following specialists should be considered for aggressive palliative interventions:

- senior palliative medicine specialist for the assessment and evaluation of particularly complex situations and recommendations for aggressive interventions
- radiation oncologist for a limited course of palliative radiation therapy
- neurosurgeon for spinal implantation of drug-infusion systems or neurological ablation
- anesthesiologist for nerve blocks, epidural, or intrathecal infusion of opioids and adjuvant drugs
- medical oncologist for palliative chemotherapy

- orthopedic surgeon for bone stabilization
- psychiatrist for management of severe depression or delirium
- grief counselor, senior hospice chaplain, clergy, or spiritual adviser for investigation of remorse or fear; loss of meaning; family of origin issues; or unresolved guilt.

Suicide in the Terminally Ill and Elderly

The prevalence of suicidal ideation and suicide attempts in the terminally ill population has not been widely studied. However, evidence suggests that vulnerability to suicide increases in patients who have a serious illness with a poor prognosis and depression.[14] The age group with the highest risk of suicide is the elderly.[70] The demographics of those with the highest risk factors for suicide include older age, male gender, white race, and single status. The risk of committing suicide for a white American man over the age of 65 is five times higher than the general US population.[70]

In many cases, a patient's request for assisted suicide or euthanasia results from uncontrolled pain and psychosocial or spiritual concerns such as loneliness and isolation, concerns about being a burden, loss of purpose, and a sense of meaninglessness. When effective, comprehensive palliative interventions such as pain and symptom relief, emotional support, and skilled interventions to alleviate spiritual pain are provided, requests for assisted suicide usually abate, and patients begin viewing life as worth living until death occurs.[71]

In a 16-month study of 988 terminally ill patients, 60.2% supported euthanasia or physician-assisted suicide in a hypothetical situation but only 10.6% reported considering either intervention for themselves.[72] During the course of the study, half of the patients who had considered either euthanasia or physician-assisted suicide for themselves changed their minds and decided against either one, and an almost equal number began considering the interventions for themselves, particularly patients with depressive symptoms, dyspnea, and substantial caregiving needs.

A patient's desire for assisted suicide or euthanasia should prompt immediate, empathetic inquiries about the presence of uncontrolled physical symptoms and psychological and spiritual pain, followed by skilled interventions designed to alleviate all sources of distress. **Table 23** describes factors associated with increased risk of suicide in patients with advanced disease.

Psychiatric hospitalization or restraints are not the best options for terminally ill patients who are contemplating suicide. Instead, appropriate interventions in the home or a palliative care inpatient setting are more likely to be helpful to the patient and family. The following are goals of intervention[14,71]:

- Prevent suicides resulting from uncontrolled physical symptoms, isolation, a sense of meaninglessness, fears of being a burden, and other conditions that often can be alleviated.
- Relieve suffering caused by treatable physical conditions.
- Provide caring presence and supportive counseling to help alleviate psychological and spiritual pain.
- Arrange for religious rites and rituals to help alleviate distress, if desired by the patient.

When unrelieved suffering continues despite expert intervention by the entire team and appropriate specialists, patients may request physician-assisted suicide. Some physicians believe this can be an appropriate and humane response to unrelieved suffering in carefully selected cases and with adequate safeguards; others object to physician-assisted suicide on religious, moral, and professional grounds. (See UNIPAC 6.) Regardless of personal beliefs, physicians can continue working to alleviate the patient's distress and prevent feelings of abandonment.[73]

Palliative Sedation

Patients at the end of life or those with refractory symptoms of shortness of breath or pain should not be left

---

Table 23. Risk Factors for Suicide in Patients with Advanced Disease

Related to Disease

Uncontrolled pain

Advanced disease and poor prognosis

Pharyngeal, lung, gastrointestinal, urogenital, or breast cancer

Advanced HIV disease

Exhaustion and fatigue

Related to Mental Status

Depression and hopelessness

Delirium and disinhibition

Psychotic features (hallucinations and delusions)

Loss of control and impulsiveness

Irrational thinking

Persistent suicidal ideation and lethal plans

Related to Personal and Family History

Preexisting psychiatric disease (major depression, anxiety disorders)

Substance abuse (alcohol)

Recent loss (spouse or friends)

Lack of social supports

Older age, male sex

Prior suicide attempts and family history of suicide

Severe existential distress

Fears of being a burden

---

to suffer. These patients should be offered palliative sedation as a therapeutic option. Palliative sedation uses sedative medications to bring comfort and treat refractory and severe symptoms of suffering. The patient is rendered unconscious and the normal process of death is allowed to take place. The sedative medication is titrated to comfort. The use of this treatment option is not intended to hasten death. The following are examples of sedative medications:

- midazolam, 0.5 mg to 3.0 mg every hour by SC or IV infusion (can be combined with morphine), titrated to relief of distress or unconsciousness
- lorazepam, 0.5 mg to 1.0 mg per hour by IV or SC infusion, titrated to relief of distress
- phenobarbital, 130 mg SC hourly until calm, and then by SC infusion (600-1,200 mg/day)[74]
- thiopental, 20 mg to 200 mg per hour, or methohexital continuous IV infusion titrated to unconsciousness.[75]

CLINICAL SITUATION

John and Tanya

John, a 36-year-old man, is between jobs (a common state for him) when he is diagnosed with colon cancer. Because he has always been suspicious of authority and bureaucracy, John insists on doing things his own way and refuses to keep his chemotherapy appointments. John self-medicates his discomfort with alcohol and heroin until the disease becomes quite advanced.

As John's disease progresses and the small amounts of heroin he can afford to buy lose their effectiveness, his extreme pain becomes frightening and he asks his girlfriend, Tanya, to help him commit suicide with the remaining drugs. Tanya wants to help John, but she is frightened and has misgivings about helping her longtime boyfriend commit suicide. She also fears that John's situation will worsen if the suicide attempt fails.

Tanya doesn't know what to do and frantically calls the oncologist for help. The oncologist says nothing more can be done for John and suggests hospice care. As John's suffering increases, Tanya calls the hospice program despite John's protests. She talks with the admission staff, thinking that the program might help John end his own life—an event Tanya now supports but with which she does not want to be personally involved.

Question One

When the hospice physician meets with John and Tanya, which of the following is the most appropriate response?

A. Reassure John that suicide can be successfully accomplished, and explain how he can overdose on heroin.

B. Prescribe 100 secobarbital capsules and tell John not to take all of them at once or he will die.

C. Help John identify childhood problems that led to fears of authority.

D. Begin aggressive treatment of John's pain, nausea, and existential distress; explore pertinent clinical, biographical, and cultural facts; and offer John admission to a hospice and palliative care inpatient unit if one is available.

Correct Response and Analysis

A is incorrect. Although John (and perhaps the physician) may believe this response is correct, in most cases relieving distressing physical symptoms and providing caring and nonjudgmental presence helps patients find a reason to live and requests for assisted suicide cease. B is incorrect because it is illegal and premature. C is incorrect because patients are unlikely to focus on psychological or spiritual issues until their physical symptoms are relieved.

D is the correct response. More information is needed before making any decisions about interventions. The simple maneuver of completing a history and physical is most likely to reveal information about John's physical, psychological, and spiritual pain. A hospice and palliative care inpatient unit is likely the best setting for initiating management of John's symptoms, but the symptoms can be managed at home.

The Case Continues

In the hospice and palliative care inpatient unit, a rapid but careful history and physical exam reveal a desperate 36-year-old man whose principal complaint is severe abdominal pain. John has not had a bowel movement for 7 days and has vomited up all food for the past 2 days. John's physical exam reveals needle tracks on his arms and a massively distended, firm abdomen with some high-pitched bowel sounds.

John is given hydromorphone by SC infusion, and the dosage is rapidly escalated until some relief is obtained despite his high tolerance for opioids. Other medications are added, and the infusion is adjusted several times a day for the next 3 days until John stabilizes on hydromorphone, 300 mg daily; haloperidol, 10 mg daily; and midazolam, 20 mg daily.

Enemas and oral sorbitol (20 mL three times per day) finally result in bowel movements, which bring considerable relief. John is now able to eat a moderate amount of food without nausea and can walk for short distances. He uses a wheelchair to make frequent visits to the garden located outside the inpatient facility, and he enjoys visits from his friends.

Tanya is greatly relieved to see John becoming more comfortable. She talks at length with the social worker and chaplain about her life with John and his illness. Although John is less willing to talk, he spends some time with the social worker and voices some regret about his alienation from his family and the way he has spent the past 15 years. He no longer mentions suicide.

As soon as his physical symptoms are relieved, John is convinced that he can return home and get back on his feet, but his strength begins to wane and his bowels stop responding to vigorous laxative regimens. Attempts to reach John's family are unsuccessful. Tanya does not believe she can care for John by herself after he becomes bed bound. John rarely talks about going home.

After 2 weeks in the hospice inpatient unit, John requires approximately 500 mg of SC hydromorphone daily in addition to the SC haloperidol, 10 mg per day; hydroxyzine, 75 mg per day (added to control nausea and itching); and midazolam, 25 mg per day for nausea and anxiety. He sleeps a great deal and is becoming more confused.

One morning John awakens and insists on going home, but he won't say why. Tanya and John's friends are afraid he will kill himself with street drugs and try to persuade him to remain in the inpatient unit, but John is determined to go home.

Question Two

At this point, which of the following is the most appropriate response for the hospice team?

A. Because of concerns about possible suicide attempts, refuse to continue caring for John, remove the SC infusion, and discharge John to his home.
B. Transfer John to a locked psychiatric facility to prevent him from harming himself.
C. Honor John's request after reaching mutually agreed upon parameters for reasonable safety.
D. Sedate John with intramuscular chlorpromazine so he will forget his request.

Correct Response and Analysis

A is incorrect for several reasons, including the return of severe pain that will occur if the infusion is removed. B is incorrect because it will be more difficult to ensure John will receive adequate symptom control in a psychiatric facility and, at this point, there is no indication that John is intent on committing suicide.

C is the correct response. The principle of patient autonomy supports honoring a patient's request, even when the physician disagrees with the patient's decision. However, the physician also has a professional duty to avoid harming the patient. Because John has not mentioned suicide and no longer seems depressed, the physician is willing to work with John and Tanya to develop a plan that satisfies John's need to return home but also honors the physician's concerns about John's safety.

D is incorrect because it ignores John's wishes and the principle of patient autonomy, which supports John's right to participate in decisions about his care as long as he is able.

The Case Concludes

John is unwilling to talk about what he wants to do while he is at home, but he continues to insist that he has to go. The physician is concerned about John's safety, but John has not mentioned suicide recently, does not seem depressed, and promises to not kill himself. With some reluctance, and after John agrees to return to the unit and allow Tanya and a friend to accompany him home, the physician agrees to a 4-hour pass. The physician teaches Tanya to operate the SC syringe driver in case John experiences increased pain.

While at home John makes decisions about his personal belongings and teaches his friend to care for his pet iguana. John returns willingly to the hospice and palliative care inpatient unit, where he soon lapses into a deep sleep and dies peacefully 2 days later.

CLINICAL SITUATION

Ms. Clarke

Ms. Clarke is a 75-year-old woman with advanced amyotrophic lateral sclerosis (ALS) who is living in a nursing home, where she receives feedings through a gastrostomy tube. Because Ms. Clarke's condition has recently deteriorated, she is referred to a hospice and palliative care program by her attending physician. Upon admitting her to the program, the team discovers that Ms. Clarke's attending physician has written standing orders for IM injections of diazepam to be given whenever Ms. Clarke awakens. When asked about the orders, the physician replies that they comply with Ms. Clarke's wishes to remain asleep until she dies. The program's medical director is disturbed by the patient's apparent poor quality of life and wonders if there isn't a better way to help Ms. Clarke.

Question One

What is the most effective intervention at this time?
A. Discontinue the IM injections of diazepam immediately.
B. Request team and family meetings to evaluate Ms. Clarke's situation.
C. Continue the injections as ordered.
D. Ignore the situation because the attending physician is caring for the patient.

Correct Response and Analysis

A is incorrect because it ignores professional etiquette and may be premature.

B is the correct response. More information is needed before any decisions are made about medication orders. Because Ms. Clarke is almost unable to speak, discussing her situation with her family, friends, other team members, and the attending physician is the best way to obtain important information. Involving other team members in Ms. Clarke's care is the best way to ensure that her physical, social, psychological, and spiritual needs are met.

C and D are incorrect because they are unlikely to reduce the suffering that Ms. Clarke may be experiencing.

The Case Continues

During the team and family meetings, the following facts emerge.

Clinical Facts
- Ms. Clarke's condition is deteriorating, and she is having more difficulty moving her facial muscles.
- Before the initiation of the diazepam IM injections, Ms. Clarke used a communicator board to express feelings of isolation and depression.

Biographical Facts
- Ms. Clarke's brother also had ALS, and he died an agonizing death by choking as the family watched helplessly.
- Ms. Clarke is haunted by the memory of her brother's terrible death and is so fearful of a similar fate that she has asked her physician to allow her to sleep until she dies.
- Ms. Clarke was married for a brief time but has been single for years.
- Ms. Clarke devoted her life to her career as a hospital administrator.
- Ms. Clarke's only relatives are two nephews of whom she is very fond, but they live out of town and can visit only periodically.
- Because the injections keep Ms. Clarke asleep almost all the time, her friends and nephews have stopped visiting her.

Other Facts

- The hospice executive director previously worked as a hospital administrator and has access to directories of hospital administrators.
- Some team members believe they should honor Ms. Clarke's expressed wish to sleep until she dies.
- The hospice gets regular referrals from the attending physician and wants to avoid angering him.

Question Two

Which of the following is the most appropriate response at this time?

A. The hospice physician will discuss the medical aspects of Ms. Clarke's care with the attending physician.
B. The executive director will try to locate information about Ms. Clarke in the directory of hospital administrators.
C. The social worker will contact Ms. Clarke's nephews to ask for more information about their aunt and for permission to begin a trial of decreased sedation if the attending physician agrees. The social worker will also request that the nephews visit their aunt.
D. As soon as Ms. Clarke awakens, the nurse will notify the hospice chaplain so a pastoral visit can be offered.
E. All the above

Correct Response and Analysis

The correct answer is E. By involving the entire team in Ms. Clarke's care, it is more likely that effective interventions will relieve her apparent psychological and spiritual distress.

The Case Continues

Although some members of the team and Ms. Clarke's attending physician want to honor her request to sleep, they agree to a short trial of decreased sedation if Ms. Clarke consents and does not appear to be in distress. Instead of using diazepam IM injections, lower doses of lorazepam will be put in her gastrostomy tube so she will be more alert. The team agrees that, in the event Ms. Clarke experiences overwhelming anxiety while awake, sedation will be restarted using medications delivered by less painful routes than IM injections.

The executive director finds a directory entry describing Ms. Clarke's career. She began working in the 1940s and received several awards during the many years she worked as an administrator. The social worker makes copies of the entry and shares them with the team, including the volunteers who will be working with Ms. Clarke if she is willing to remain awake.

When the nurse alerts the chaplain (Allen) that Ms. Clarke appears to be waking up, Allen sits by her bed. He introduces himself and asks Ms. Clarke if she would stay awake for awhile because he wants to visit with her. He asks her what she thinks of his proposal. Using her communicator board, Ms. Clarke indicates she will have to think about it. She then receives another dose of lorazepam.

Later, when Ms. Clarke begins to awaken again, the hospice medical director visits with her, acknowledges her fears of choking and suffocation, and expresses dismay at her brother's terrible death. The medical director also discusses the following topics: her condition, the effects of sedation on her daily life, the tube feedings, and medications that will be used to relieve distressing symptoms should they occur. The medical director again reassures Ms. Clarke that the hospice and palliative care team and her attending physicians will work together to make sure her symptoms are controlled. The medical director also expresses the wish that Ms. Clarke will decide to stay awake during the day so she can visit with people and experience some enjoyment in her life. Ms. Clarke's eyes tear up and she indicates that she will think about it.

The following morning Allen visits again, this time with the paper describing Ms. Clarke's career. Finding Ms. Clarke drowsy but easily aroused, Allen dangles the paper in front of her. "Well, I found out you are quite a woman! According to this, you were running an entire hospital during a time most women were hardly allowed out of the house!" Ms. Clarke's eyes light up and Allen continues talking for a few minutes. "You are really something! Just think of all the people you touched during your career. You helped saved a lot of lives and you made it possible for people to keep their jobs at the hospital. You were quite an administrator. Look what it says here." Allen then reads the description to Ms. Clarke and asks her some questions about her life as a young woman. Ms. Clarke indicates she would like to keep the paper by her bed, and her expression is animated as Allen comments on her various awards and achievements.

In the meantime, the social worker talks with Ms. Clarke's nephews, who describe their aunt's favorite music and books, mention an album of old photographs they have, and agree to visit that weekend. The next time Ms. Clarke awakens, the social worker visits with her, tells her about her nephews' plan to visit, and asks if she would like to listen to some of the music that they recommended. Ms. Clarke agrees and seems contented for several hours. A volunteer visits and offers to read to her, and Ms. Clarke indicates she would enjoy listening to a book of short stories.

Ms. Clarke decides to try a course of decreased sedation in the hope she will be able to visit with her nephews when they arrive, and her attending physician agrees. The nurse titrates the lorazepam as ordered and assures Ms. Clarke that her medication will be increased immediately if she even looks like she might be having difficulty breathing. Because Ms. Clarke is now more awake, hospice staff and volunteers drop in frequently to say hello.

When her nephews visit, they reminisce about the times Ms. Clarke took them to ball games at Yankee Stadium and laugh about old times. They also look at the photograph album the social worker suggested they bring with them.

For 2 weeks Ms. Clarke's quality of life is much improved, and she no longer asks for lorazepam during the day. Then she vomits some of the tube feedings. Despite quick suctioning and a decreased rate of tube feeding, it becomes clear that aspiration pneumonitis is resulting in shortness of breath.

Question Three

Which is the best intervention at this time? (Choose all that apply.)

A. Order an increased dose of lorazepam.
B. Transfer Ms.Clarke to an acute-care setting for intravenous antibiotic treatment.
C. Suggest that the attending physician order a subcutaneous infusion of morphine and midazolam.
D. Increase the number of visits by volunteers and staff.

Correct Response and Analysis

A is incorrect because lorazepam alone is less likely to alleviate her cough and dyspnea. B is incorrect because treating the pneumonia will only ensure that, if she lives a few days longer, Ms. Clarke will be in an isolated environment. In the past, Ms. Clarke indicated she did not want interventions that would prolong her increasing, severe disability.

C and D are the correct responses. An SC infusion of morphine and midazolam is easier to titrate and more humane than IM injections of diazepam and is much more likely to control Ms. Clarke's anxiety and any pain and breathlessness she may experience. Increased visits by volunteers and staff will also reduce her anxiety and her sense of isolation.

The Case Concludes

When Ms. Clarke's symptoms worsen, the morphine is increased to 30 mg per day and the midazolam to 10 mg per day. Because the tube feedings are likely to be increasing her distressing pulmonary secretions and are serving only to prolong the dying process, they are discontinued with permission from Ms. Clarke, her attending physician, and her nephews. Before discontinuing the treatment, the nursing home staff is educated about the benefits and burdens of artificial nutrition in this particular situation. The reasons for discontinuing a now burdensome procedure are also explained.

Ms. Clarke remains calm and drowsy but is able to respond to her nephews and her close friends. Two days later, Ms. Clarke dies a peaceful death in the nursing home surrounded by hospice staff and the volunteers who have stayed by her bedside for most of the day. After Ms. Clarke dies, her nephews thank the physician and the hospice for their interventions and indicate that the final few weeks of their aunt's life had been the most rewarding since she became ill.

Social Pain

Considering the burdens of terminal illness on patients, families, and caregivers, the interdisciplinary team must comprehensively assess social supports and stressors. Chronic or terminal illnesses can result in social isolation through the loss of physical function, alterations in body image, or illness-related disfigurement. In addition, the physical and emotional demands of caregiving can be stressful on a family unit or other care providers as well as disrupt normal family dynamics. Caring for family members with chronic or terminal disease can also have significant negative financial effects.

Caregiving

Caring for a patient with a terminal illness is an extremely stressful process. There are an estimated 44.4 million caregivers in the United States, with most end-of-life care provided in patients' homes. The primary caregiver is most often the spouse, followed by an adult child. The majority of caregivers are women, and many do not live with the patient. Caregivers spend an average of 20.5 hours per week providing care, and 20% of caregivers spend more than 40 hours per week caring for a person at home. Caregivers may be expected to provide a range of support for patients, including the provision of activities of daily living (bathing, dressing, and hygiene), care of medical problems, medication management, wound care, and much more. Caregivers may feel poorly prepared to take on these tasks.[76,77] Because of differences in caregivers' socioeconomic status, minority caregivers may have more unmet needs and may provide higher levels of care.[78]

The Stress Process Model shown in **Figure 2** serves as a framework to understand the dimensions of caregiving in palliative and end-of-life care.[79] The model incorporates primary and secondary stressors as well as resources to improve caregiver stress.

The Caregiver-Patient Relationship

Schulz and colleagues propose a conceptual model of caregiving that links patient suffering and caregiver compassion. In this framework, patient suffering has physical, psychological, and existential manifestations. The compassion the caregiver feels for the patient is moderated by factors such as empathy, proximity, and quality of the relationship. In addition to the relationship between suffering and compassion, patient suffering may have a direct effect on physical and emotional outcomes in the caregiver.[80]

Consequences of Caregiving

Caregiving can result in significant emotional and physical distress for the caregiver. **Table 24** lists some common negative consequences of caregiving. Providing care prevents many people from engaging in their own interests, normal activities, socialization, and employment.[81] In addition, caregiving for patients with terminal illness can result in significant financial strain. In 20% of families, caregivers had to stop working, and 31% of families lost their savings during a loved one's terminal illness.[82]

Caregiving may also present significant psychological burdens. Caregivers may experience emotional stress and are more likely to experience depression, anxiety, and other general psychiatric symptoms.[82] This is especially true for caregivers of persons with dementia.[83,84]

Treatment and Resources for Caregivers

Assessing and treating caregiver burdens require the full effort of the interdisciplinary team. Caregivers' needs may shift significantly as patients transition through their illness, from diagnosis and the initiation of caregiving through death, bereavement, and the disengagement of the caregiving role.[85]

The patient's illness may also affect the caregiving experience. Three basic illness trajectories are gradual decline (dementia or stroke), progressive illness with a short terminal phase (cancer), and gradual decline with multiple episodes of acute illness (congestive heart failure, HIV/AIDS, lung disease). Each trajectory presents unique challenges to the caregiver.[78]

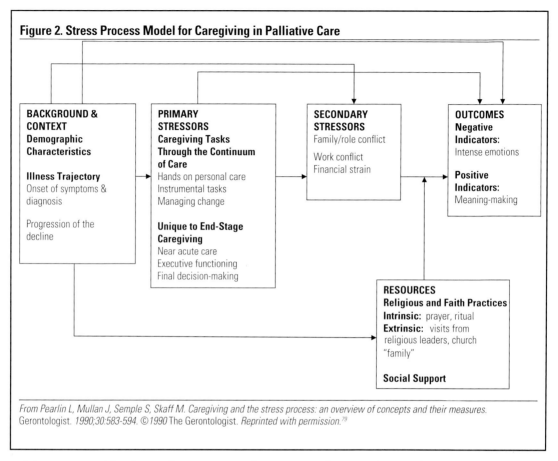

Figure 2. Stress Process Model for Caregiving in Palliative Care

BACKGROUND & CONTEXT
Demographic Characteristics

Illness Trajectory
Onset of symptoms & diagnosis

Progression of the decline

PRIMARY STRESSORS
Caregiving Tasks Through the Continuum of Care
Hands on personal care
Instrumental tasks
Managing change

Unique to End-Stage Caregiving
Near acute care
Executive functioning
Final decision-making

SECONDARY STRESSORS
Family/role conflict
Work conflict
Financial strain

OUTCOMES
Negative Indicators:
Intense emotions

Positive Indicators:
Meaning-making

RESOURCES
Religious and Faith Practices
Intrinsic: prayer, ritual
Extrinsic: visits from religious leaders, church "family"

Social Support

From Pearlin L, Mullan J, Semple S, Skaff M. Caregiving and the stress process: an overview of concepts and their measures. Gerontologist. *1990;30:583-594.* © *1990* The Gerontologist. *Reprinted with permission.*[79]

Primary care providers for caregivers must remember to consider caregiving burdens and keep in mind that physical symptoms may be manifestations of caregiver stress. In addition, although women are more likely to be caregivers, men are less likely to seek help for certain problems and are more vulnerable to physiologic distress caused by caregiving. Persons with lower educational levels (less than high school) and older caregivers are at increased risk for emotional distress caused by caregiving. Caregivers who are able to maintain employment may be at lower risk for caregiver stress.[83] Despite the negative aspects of caregiving, providing care for a loved one with advanced illness may be a very rewarding experience. **Table 25** lists some of the positive aspects of caregiving.

Important strategies to help caregivers include providing education and information, providing assistance with care, and encouraging caregivers to continue to engage in activities they value. Caregivers may need training and education about a patient's illness, what symptoms to expect, and specific care needs of the patient. Caregivers should also be informed about the potential for caregiver stress and its consequences as well as strategies to relieve stress. These include increased reliance on other family members to help with care, participation in support groups, and maintaining activities they value, when possible. Patients and families may benefit from increased assistance with care, whether the assistance comes from government-sponsored home care programs, volunteer programs (especially those provided in hospice care), adult day programs, or the use of respite care. Individual and family counseling and information about grief and loss should be offered.[83]

Table 24. Negative Consequences of Caregiving
Loss of normal family roles
Increased social isolation
Decrease in normal social activities
Inability to continue regular employment
Financial strain
Depression
Anxiety
Psychiatric complaints
Physical burdens or symptoms
Increased risk of mortality
Loss of intimacy

Table 25. Positive Aspects of Caregiving[83]
Pride in being able to provide care
Increased self-efficacy or self-worth
Strengthening of personal relationships
Personal or spiritual growth
Increased meaning

Religion may also play an important role in caregiving. A study of 1,229 caregivers of family members with dementia examined the relationship between religion and mental health.[86] The results demonstrated that religious beliefs were upheld and important to many caregivers, and religious practice and adherence to traditions were associated with less clinical depression.

Complicated Grief

Complicated grief involves grief that is complicated by the development of adjustment disorders, depression, anxiety, or substance abuse. Approximately 10% to 20% of people will experience a period of prolonged and pathologic grief known as complicated grief.[87] Complicated grief may be associated with a prolonged duration of often exaggerated symptoms and a disruption of normal function and social relationships and occurs for 6 months or longer after death. Worden identified four types of complicated grief: chronic, delayed, masked, and exaggerated. See **Table 26** for the definitions of the four types of complicated grief and their associated symptoms.

Assessment

Unless physicians get to know the person who is experiencing a loss, they are unlikely to intervene effectively.[8] Instead of relieving suffering, a physician may unwittingly exacerbate the patient's or family member's anguish by suggesting psychiatric referrals and prescribing pharmacological therapy when education, interpretation, compassionate communication, and ongoing emotional support are more appropriate interventions. Before attempting to assess and manage complicated grief, clinicians should become familiar with the common reactions to loss listed in Table 14 (page 26).

In most cases mourners realize they are experiencing problems with the grieving process and ask healthcare professionals for help. When people who experience traumatic losses do not recognize that their otherwise unexplainable medical or psychiatric problems are likely associated with unresolved grief, their grief-related problems (often anxiety and depression) often compel them to visit a physician. Considerable skill is then required to reveal unacknowledged losses.[43,88]

Management

Attempts to short-circuit grief are not only inappropriate, they are certain to fail. When patients and families allow themselves to feel the deep pain of loss, they are more likely to experience eventual healing. By normalizing common reactions to loss, physicians can provide family members with a foundation for healing; however, after particularly distressing deaths, the grieving process may be protracted. Shear concluded that complicated grief needs early intervention by a mental health professional.[89] The incorporation of a targeted complicated grief treatment over routine interpersonal psychotherapy was associated with improved rates of response.[90]

Resisting the temptation to offer simplistic solutions for complex problems is an important part of the intervention process. For example, immediately prescribing medications to relieve the distressing symptoms of grief (sadness, insomnia, anxiety) without fully investigating

Table 26. Four Types of Complicated Grief[43]

Chronic Grief

Definition: Continuance of acute grief reaction over a prolonged period of time (usually defined as 6 months after death).

Chronic grief may indicate the mourner is stuck; the process of grieving has halted.
- Grief is static (ie, the levels of depression, anger, or guilt remain unchanged for months or years).
- The patient has a long history of unexplained pain, depression, and/or anxiety that began with the loss of a loved one.

Delayed Grief

Definition: Bereavement occurring years or decades after a loss.

Mourners may attempt to delay grief when losses have overwhelmed their ability to cope. Delayed grief is most common when a death is completely unexpected, particularly violent, or the result of suicide or a criminal act.
- Expressions of grief are suppressed or inhibited.
- Minor events trigger intense reactions even years after the death.
- Responses to a recent death seem out of proportion to the degree of loss.
- Mourners are unable to talk about the deceased without fresh expressions of grief even many years after the death.

Masked Grief

Definition: A condition in which symptoms of grief may be absent or appear unrelated to the loss.

Masked grief is likely when mourners develop the following symptoms and are unable to recognize them as related to grief:
- avoidance of any emotion when discussing either the deceased or the bereaved's current situation
- unexplained anxiety and depression
- aberrant or maladaptive behaviors (eg, an inability to leave the house or panic attacks)
- disabling, nonaffective physical symptoms similar to those experienced by the deceased (ie, pain, nausea, numbness, anorexia)
- chronic changes in lifestyle following a death (eg, withdrawal from friends)
- avoidance of the grave site, nonparticipation in death-related rituals such as funerals, unwillingness to read cards of condolence, chronic unwillingness to move any of the deceased's material possessions
- self-destructive behaviors (eg, failure to provide for basic survival needs such as safety and nutrition and abuse of alcohol or prescription drugs).

Exaggerated Grief

Definition: Grief characterized by excessive and disabling symptoms that may worsen with time.

Unlike masked grief, when mourners are unaware their symptoms are related to grief, exaggerated grief is more likely when mourners understand their symptoms are related to grief, they feel completely overwhelmed for long periods of time by conditions such as the following:
- depression and/or anxiety
- a severe inability to concentrate
- feelings of helplessness and hopelessness
- feelings of worthlessness and emptiness
- irrational despair
- panic attacks
- phobias about illness or death
- mania
- persistent thoughts of suicide or forming a plan to commit suicide.

associated psychological, physical, social, and spiritual factors is unlikely to be helpful over the long run. Medications can mask or temporarily relieve the symptoms of unresolved grief, but they cannot alleviate the underlying condition. Unless anxiety or depressive symptoms are interfering significantly with daily functioning or the mourner's ability to negotiate the grieving process, medications should be avoided or used sparingly.

Resilience after traumatic loss is common and occurs on a trajectory distinct from that of the recovery process. Many people continue to have positive experiences even after serious loss or trauma.[91] See the section "Anxiety and Depression" on page 28.

The following interventions are likely to help prevent or resolve complicated grief[43]:

- Rule out physical disease.
- Assess for risk factors that predict complicated grief reactions (see **Table 27**).
- Normalize the grieving process (eg, provide education about common reactions to loss).
- Help the bereaved identify all the losses they have experienced as a result of the patient's illness and death and other, previous losses.[87]
- Validate the pain of grief and help the bereaved identify and express their grief-related reactions.
- Provide ongoing support during the grieving process and monitor the bereaved's progress.
- Employ the skills and resources of an interdisciplinary team, including a chaplain, social worker, and counselor, and refer when needed to
  - a hospice bereavement program or support group such as Compassionate Friends or another appropriate psychoeducational bereavement support group[92]
  - mental health professionals with special training in grief therapy (eg, grief therapists, specialized psychiatrists)
  - a physician for short-term drug therapy for disabling anxiety and depression
  - assessment for suicide ideation. taking appropriate measures when necessary.

Physicians and Personal Stress

Dr. Cicely Saunders recognized the possibilities for mutual growth when she suggested that a dying patient needs the community and the community needs the dying patient. As dying patients search for renewed purpose and hope, they are likely to inspire hospice and palliative medicine physicians and others to engage in their own search for meaning and to explore their own sources of meaning.

The opportunities for developing the insight and wisdom that occur when working with dying patients can help physicians provide better care for all patients and their family members. Physicians also are likely to learn methods for coping with the inevitable psychological and spiritual pain that will occur in their own lives. Few professional opportunities offer such great rewards.

When caring for dying patients, physicians need to acknowledge their own needs and anticipate the occurrence of psychological and spiritual issues that will inevitably cause them personal distress.[93] The recommendations listed in **Table 28** are likely to help physicians maintain their personal equilibrium while continuing to grow both personally and professionally. (For more specific information about coping with personal stress, see UNIPAC 5.)

Initially a patient's psychological and spiritual issues that arise during the course of a terminal illness may appear hopelessly complicated or entrenched in a patient's and family's lifelong patterns of dysfunctional coping. However, a caring presence and appropriate interventions can alleviate much of the pain caused by psychological and spiritual concerns. The pressures of daily practice can make the provision of such interventions difficult, but it is possible for physicians to care for patients and families in ways that are life enhancing for all concerned.

Table 27. Risk Factors for Complicated Grief[43]

What the Loss Was and Who the Deceased Person Was
Reactions to loss vary depending on the particular meaning of the loss for a specific person. Because a terminal illness often means the approaching loss of everything a dying patient has ever known and cared about, reactions can be severe. Conjugal losses generally lead to protracted disorganization, while the loss of a child may evoke the most lasting and intense yearning and anger. The age of the deceased also affects the bereaved person's reactions to loss; the death of a child generally is associated with complicated grief.

Nature of the Attachment
Clinging or ambivalent relationships are associated with complicated grief, particularly when initial feelings of relief are followed by feelings of anger and guilt. Difficult grief reactions may occur when the deceased was the survivor's primary source of self-worth and self-esteem (eg, when a dependent partner dies, the survivor may have difficulty finding a role to replace the one of caretaker).

Mode of Loss or Death
Losses, including deaths, that are sudden, unexpected, untimely, and multiple are more likely to result in complicated grief. Deaths associated with suicide, mutilation, or perceived threats to the survivor's life typically result in patterns of grieving characterized by attempts to avoid, repress, or delay grief for months or years at a time. The numbness associated with the normal process of grieving may persist for long periods of time. Attempts to delay grief will not prevent the bereaved from experiencing high levels of ongoing anger and tension.

Historical Antecedents
Previous patterns of coping may predict responses to a loss, but successful integration of expected and timely losses may not predict reactions to unexpected, violent losses.

A history of psychiatric illness, including major depression or anxiety disorders, increases the risk of a difficult grieving process. Past or current threats of suicide are associated with complicated grief.

Multiple losses can result in chronic serial grief, a devastating condition that results from the loss of several significant relationships, one soon after another.

Personality Variables
Past or current misuse of alcohol or other drugs and tendencies to depression and anxiety are associated with a difficult grieving process, as are difficulties coping with stress or a lack of trust in self and others.

Social Factors
Frequent moves, estrangement, geographical separation from other family members, and lack of supportive networks such as church or social groups can adversely affect the grieving process. The presence of caring family members who provide support for those most affected by the loss is often a predictor of good outcome.

A lack of cultural norms with established models for mourning can adversely affect the grieving process.

Concurrent Stressors
Losses that result in major life changes, such as serious economic reversals, moves, job changes, and abrupt changes in caregiving responsibilities for young children often affect the grieving process adversely.

Table 28. Managing Stress in Palliative Care

Acknowledge the likelihood of periodic challenges to the clinician's own psychological and spiritual equilibrium.

Recognize the clinician's own limitations and the inability to ensure a perfect outcome for every patient and family.

Recognize that skillfully using available knowledge, treatments, and resources; providing a caring presence; and involving team members and consultants is all that can be done.

Balance work, home life, and leisure activities to avoid exhaustion and burnout.

Get adequate rest and take as many vacations as possible.

Use religious and/or spiritual practices to strengthen the clinician's own inner resources.

Discuss painful psychological and spiritual issues with others (eg, interested peers, clergy, counselors).

Locate resources for assistance with difficult cases. Call AAHPM for help locating other hospice and palliative care physicians and attend palliative medicine conferences.

Spiritual Pain

Spiritual Care

Healthcare providers will encounter numerous situations involving varying degrees of spiritual healing, hope, and remorse. Spiritual care is an integral part of each interdisciplinary team member's domain of caring, and each member can provide spiritual care at some level.

Regardless of discipline, requirements for providing spiritual care include the following skills:

- knowledge of the fundamental principles of spiritual care, common spiritual concerns, indicators of spiritual pain, interventions to alleviate spiritual pain, and the core beliefs and practices of major religions; spiritual pain should not be overlooked or disregarded in patients without a religious denomination
- active listening, empathetic communication, and identifying the spiritual issues embedded in a patient's stories of the past and present
- presence, including the ability to remain present and available as patients and families explore troubling spiritual issues and search for renewed meaning
- intuition based on knowledge, skills, and presence and acceptance of the universally pervasive mysteries of human existence that transcend culture and religion.

Physicians specializing in hospice and palliative medicine should be able to assess for the presence of spiritual pain and provide basic interventions. A study of 248 patients that assessed the nature of dying patients' spiritual needs demonstrated that those near the end of life wanted to communicate about fear, hope, and spirituality. The study revealed that 45% of patients who had no religious denomination wanted their physicians to approach the subject of spirituality.[94]

However, before attempting to personally address complicated spiritual pain, physicians should consider several issues. Alleviating complicated spiritual pain requires knowledge, skills, and time for unhurried reflection. Alleviating complicated spiritual pain also requires the skills and resources of an entire interdisciplinary team of healthcare professionals. If an interdisciplinary care team is not available, will the physician be able to involve other disciplines, including pastoral caregivers, therapists, and grief counselors? Also, physicians should be aware that additional training is needed to alleviate complicated spiritual pain. The assumption that anyone with interest and common sense can effectively intervene in cases of complicated spiritual pain trivializes this type of pain and is likely to result in less than optimal care.[95] Ongoing training sessions must be available for physicians and other members of the healthcare team.

Universal Spiritual Concerns

Regardless of their religious affiliation or lack thereof, people deal with universal spiritual issues when they try to make sense of existence, suffering, and death. Questions such as the following indicate a patient (or physician) is grappling with spiritual or religious concerns:

- Why am I here? Does life have any meaning?
- Are people part of something larger than themselves?
- Does a higher power such as God exist; if so, what is my relationship to that power?
- Why do people suffer? Why must I suffer?
- Is suffering a punishment for something? Am I to blame?
- Are people at fault for the suffering of their loved ones? Did I cause my loved one's suffering?
- Does death have any meaning? Do people live and die for nothing?
- What happens after people die?

Theoretical Frameworks for Understanding Spirituality

Religion is an interconnection of sacred texts, customs, and beliefs adopted by a community. Spirituality centers on an individual's interpretation and practices as a result of life questioning.[96] Although religion is often used to label groups and individuals, spirituality must be considered in a broader framework because many people do not identify with a formal religion. Spiritual issues and needs will be encountered in almost all end-of-life care. See **Table 29** for Hay's four interrelated dimensions of spiritual pain and helpful interventions. See **Table 30** for Kellehear's three dimensions of spiritual need. Both frameworks assume frequent interplay among dimensions.

Models for inclusive medical care have included the biopsychosocial model proposed by George Engel in 1977 and an ecological model introduced by White, Williams, and Greenberg in 1996.[99] Engel's model focuses on interpersonal relationships and the psychological state of the patient. The ecological model takes environmental factors into

---

Table 29. Four Interrelated Dimensions of Spiritual Pain and Helpful Interventions[97]

I. Spiritual Pain Related to Individual and Community Issues. *Spiritual development occurs within the context of the human community.*

Signs and symptoms of spiritual pain related to individual and community issues:
- Physical pain not controlled by usual means
- Torment and anguish
- Complicated reactions to loss
- Hopelessness, pervasive existential guilt
- Fear and dread
- Noncompliance with care plan
- Sense of abandonment and betrayal
- Isolation and withdrawal from support communities, breakdown of relationships

II. Spiritual Pain Related to General Issues of Meaning. *Spiritual development occurs within the context of a search for meaning.*

Signs and symptoms of spiritual pain related to issues of meaning:
- Expressions of life's meaninglessness and loss of faith
- Questioning the adequacy of present belief system, world view, or philosophy, whether religious or nonreligious
- Expressions of desire for a belief system, world view, or philosophy to help to cope with spiritual pain
- Presence of unresolved religious issues (eg, "If only I had enough faith, I would be cured").
- Guilt associated with religious beliefs
- Isolation from religious or spiritual communities with similar beliefs

Helpful interventions:
- Encourage reflection on past, current, or desired belief systems, philosophies, or world views.
- Encourage practical application of the patient's belief system or philosophy to the current situation.
- Identify elements of past or current belief system or philosophy that provided support in the past; encourage reestablishment of these elements.
- Explore the patient's religious history as a cause of pain. Some patients may feel terribly wounded by the religion of their childhood and need to come to terms with their anger and sense of rejection.
- Encourage patients to tell their life stories as a way of helping them to recognize themes of purpose, value, worth, and meaning.

III. Spiritual Pain Related to Religious Needs. *Religious beliefs shape the search for meaning; religious rites and rituals provide concrete means of expressing spirituality.*

Signs and symptoms of spiritual pain related to religious needs:
- Desire for devotional expressions of religion
- Lack of participation in religious and/or spiritual practices and rituals
- Absence of a religious leader or teacher and separation from previous religious affiliations
- Desire to practice religious and spiritual disciplines such as prayer, meditation, and yoga

continued

Table 29. Four Interrelated Dimensions of Spiritual Pain and Helpful Interventions[97] *(continued)*

Helpful interventions:
- Observe each patient's special holy days, dietary restrictions, needs for daily prayer or meditation, hygiene and modesty requirements, and other important religious precepts.
- Remember the power of religious rituals and observances and, when appropriate, provide or arrange for the following:
  - Prayers that focus on healing and reconciliation
  - The sacraments of baptism, confirmation, marriage, reconciliation, and the sacrament of the sick
  - Ritualized confession, reconciliation, absolution of sins, asking for forgiveness
  - Laying on of hands
  - Devotional practices (eg, meditation, prayer, turning toward Mecca, and reading religious scriptures from sources such as the Hebrew and Christian bibles, the Vedas, and the Koran)

IV. Spiritual Pain Related to Inner Resource Issues. *Spiritual disciplines enhance the capacity to transcend life's difficulties; they are defined as any personal practice or activity that animates, inspires, or motivates a person to aspire, hope, and participate in living. Examples include prayer, yoga, thinking, reading, walking, playing, making love, enjoying nature.*

Signs and symptoms of spiritual pain related to lack of inner resources:
- Sense of purposelessness and lack of fulfillment
- Feelings of being overwhelmed, helpless, and out of control
- Lack of awareness that anger, hurt, guilt, and fear can isolate people from their deepest selves, from others, and from ultimate reality
- Unfamiliarity with spiritual disciplines such as prayer or meditation
- Inadequate use of techniques that help people to adapt to difficult circumstances (eg, sharing feelings with others, humor, relaxation, meditation, prayer)

Helpful interventions:
- Help patients identify elements in the past that have given meaning to their lives and helped them to feel more alive and empowered (eg, use of spiritual and religious practices, contact with nature, reestablishing and enhancing relationships, meaningful communication with significant others)
- Encourage life review and exploration of sources of meaning in life.
- If the patient desires, arrange for access to books or meditation tapes to enhance inner resources.
- Encourage greater use of adaptive techniques such as relaxation, imagery, music, poetry, and devotional readings that focus on healing rather than cure. (If the patient desires, arrange for access to spiritual or religious teachers who use meditation, prayer, and religious scriptures to focus on healing instead of physical cures.)
- Help patients to reframe goals into short-term tasks that can be accomplished, such as going on a trip or saying good-bye to friends and family.

consideration. While these models have identified key relationships, both have left out the elements of spirituality.

Multidimensional, theoretical frameworks for understanding spirituality are being developed, some of which are based on a needs model. The needs model presupposes people want to find a sense of meaning that allows them to make sense of their situation and transcend their suffering.[98]

Assessment
Problems and Challenges

Alleviating spiritual pain requires careful assessment and interventions that are sometimes intensive. Most of these interventions involve empathetic presence, active listening, and continued emotional support as patients and families seek to transcend their suffering through a renewed sense of meaning. To intervene effectively, specific sources of spiritual pain should be identified. This can be difficult because of many factors. Patients

Table 30. Three Dimensions of Spiritual Need[98]

Situational Transcendence: In this dimension, patients want to make sense of and transcend their current situation. They often desire

- purpose
- hope
- meaning and affirmation
- mutuality
- a sense of connection
- social presence.

Moral and Biographical Transcendence: In this dimension, patients want to "put things right" to make sense of their own lives and to develop a sense of transcendent meaning for their existence. They often desire

- peace and reconciliation
- reunion with others
- prayer
- moral and social analysis
- forgiveness
- closure.

Religious Transcendence: In this dimension, patients want to achieve a sense of religious transcendence. They often desire

- religious reconciliation
- divine forgiveness and support
- religious rites and sacraments
- visits by clergy
- religious literature
- discussion about God, eschatology, or eternal life and hope.

rarely voice spiritual concerns until distressing physical, emotional, and social problems are alleviated.[95] Also, spiritual pain and despair frequently manifest as physical symptoms, which patients may perceive as being more acceptable to physicians. In fact, spiritual pain often shares the following features with depression: pervasive, existential guilt not connected to a particular event; feelings of hopelessness and worthlessness; and a sense of meaninglessness.

Despite these difficulties, the importance of assessing and addressing religious and spiritual well-being cannot be overstated. When assessing for the presence and sources of spiritual pain, the most effective technique is to establish a caring relationship with the patient and then simply ask about death-related concerns and beliefs. Many terminally ill patients are willing to discuss spiritual issues as long as physicians and other team members exhibit genuine interest and empathy, knowledge of spiritual concerns, effective communication skills, a nonjudgmental form of respect for the patient's beliefs, and a willingness to take the time to listen to the patient's stories as a way of exploring spiritual needs.

Special Needs of the African American Community

Special attention needs to be given to the African American population and the influence of spirituality in health care. African Americans will experience a higher burden of chronic diseases, including heart failure and diabetes. Literature has shown that African Americans are twice as likely to die from chronic or acute illness.[100]

Cultural issues, personal spirituality, and a mistrust of organized medicine all serve as barriers to high-quality end-of-life and palliative care. Compared to members of other cultures, members of the African American community are much less likely to discuss advance directives with their healthcare provider. In one study of African Americans, 75% advocated a faith-based intervention to increase advance directives. The church community is an important source of social support, health promotion, and comfort. Informal networks provided by the social structure of the church are important ways for patients to receive education and care and can be vital supplements to the palliative care team.[101]

In some cases, religious beliefs and practices contribute to spiritual pain. Examples include religious doctrines that threaten dying patients with eternal punishment for certain behaviors or beliefs. Other examples include clergy who discourage the deep spiritual questioning and exploration that usually accompany traumatic events. Some patients may be very religious, attending worship services and observing religious rituals and requirements. However, they may not be particularly spiritual (they have not yet addressed spiritual questions on a deeply personal level or developed the inner resources for coping with life's difficulties). See **Table 31** for a guide to spiritual assessment.

Ethical Issues

In 1994 only three medical schools in the United States taught courses on religious and spiritual issues. In 2004 84 schools had incorporated spirituality into the curriculum to various degrees.[102]

Despite a greater understanding of the importance of religion and spirituality in many patients' lives, particularly in the face of profound illness, the physician's role in alleviating spiritual pain remains somewhat controversial. Ethical issues may arise, particularly in the following three areas:

1. Findings are unclear whether specific religious or spiritual beliefs and practices influence health outcomes. Many patients report that their religious and spiritual beliefs and practices help them cope with their illness. Although methodological limitations of several studies made it difficult to draw conclusions, a systematic review of randomized trials of "distant healing" indicated that 57% of these trials showed a positive treatment effect, a result that merits further study.[103]

However, no universally accepted study has yet demonstrated a positive relationship between specific religious or spiritual beliefs and practices and improved health outcomes (eg, remission of advanced cancer or other terminal illness).[104] Failure to control for confounding variables, other covariates, and multiple comparisons undermines the validity of current studies and contributes to conflicting findings.[104] The absence of widely accepted definitions of *religion* and *spirituality* and *religious beliefs and practices* and *spiritual beliefs and practices* continues to undermine the validity of current studies. Until conclusive evidence is available, premature attempts to link specific religious beliefs or activities with improved health outcomes may harm patients, particularly those whose suffering is already exacerbated by a belief that their illness or lack of improvement is a result of their own moral failures, lack of faith, or lack of positive attitude. Suggesting to patients

that they should develop religious or spiritual beliefs or practices if they do not have them or desire them is inappropriate and disrespectful.[105]

2. Professional boundaries can become blurred. The physician's role in assessing for spiritual pain and referring patients for pastoral care is generally controversial. However, ethical questions may arise when physicians themselves serve as pastoral caregivers. Professional boundaries can become blurred and confusing when physicians engage in religious or spiritual practices with patients (eg, praying with patients, either at the patient's request or the physician's instigation). To avoid the perception of coercion, physician-led prayer should be avoided unless the following conditions are met[105]:

- Clergy or other pastoral caregivers are not readily available.
- The patient requests and is intent on praying with the physician.
- The physician can pray without having to feign faith.
- The physician can pray without manipulating the patient.

3. Questioning patients about their religious or spiritual beliefs is controversial. Many patients welcome physician inquiries about their spiritual or religious beliefs, particularly at the end of life. However, some patients object strongly to such inquiries. Direct, open-ended questions about religious beliefs may concern some patients, who then worry that an affirmative answer will encourage physicians to offer religious or spiritual advice.[106] This may be particularly true when the medical rationale for asking patients about their beliefs is unclear. The following questions provide a clinical rationale for questions about religious and spiritual beliefs and provide patients with a quick and unrevealing way to end such inquires if they wish to[106]:

- When dealing with a difficult situation in the past, have you relied on your spirituality for support and guidance?
- Do you have spiritual or religious beliefs that would influence your medical decisions if you become gravely ill?

Table 31. A Guide to Spiritual Assessment[96]

Assessing the Spiritual Issues Raised by Serious Illness, Especially at the End of Life
First, establish an empathic connection with the patient (or the patient's family). Often, nothing more will be required to engage the patient in significant spiritual sharing. Only then, consider moving to more specific questions.

Opening
"It must be very hard for you to find yourself (your loved one) so sick. How are you holding up?"

Questions of Meaning

Patient/family questions	*Clinician questions*
"What is the meaning of my illness?"	"Have you thought about what all this means?"
"What is the meaning of my suffering?"	"Would there be anything for which you might hope even if you (your loved one) are not cured?"
"What is the meaning of my death?"	
"Will any meaning persist beyond my death?"	"Do you attach any spiritual significance to the word 'hope'?"

Questions of Value

Patient/family questions	*Clinician questions*
"How does my value relate to my appearance?"	"Are you able to hold onto a sense of your own dignity and purpose?"
" . . . my productivity?"	"Do you feel that people in the hospital/your family/your friends/your congregation really care about you (your loved one) as a person?"
" . . . my independence?"	
"Is there anything about me that is valuable when these are threatened?"	"Are there any spiritual or religious resources upon which you can draw to help see you through this?"
"Is there anything valuable about me that will persist beyond death?"	

Questions of Relationship

Patient/family questions	*Clinician questions*
"Am I estranged from any family or friends?"	"How are things with your family and friends?"
"Who have I wronged? Who has wronged me?"	"Is there anyone with whom you need to 'make up'?"
"Am I loved? By whom?"	"Is there anyone to whom you need to say 'I love you' or 'I'm sorry'?"
"Does love endure beyond the grave?"	"If you're a religious person, how are things between you and God?"

Closing Comments
"I can't do everything—that's why we work as a team. I think we've covered some very important ground here, but there's so much more to talk about. If it's okay with you I'm going to send Rev S to see you later today. Also, I'd like to tell her a little about what you've just shared with me, so she can be better prepared. Would that be okay?"

Assessment Tools

Many spiritual assessment tools focus narrowly on religious affiliation and beliefs. They are usually based on Judeo-Christian language and presuppose a belief in God or other higher power. Other tools attempt to broaden this scope but may fail to distinguish spirituality from religion. Some tools use the terms *religious* and *spiritual* interchangeably, which undermines their validity and contributes to conflicting findings.

An example of a brief spiritual assessment tool, the FICA, is shown in **Table 32**. It was designed to be effective regardless of a patient's system of belief by helping patients voice concerns about meaning and purpose in their lives even when they fail to

Table 32. FICA: A Spiritual Assessment Tool[107]

F: Faith or Beliefs
Specific questions to elicit responses:
- Do you consider yourself spiritual or religious? Both? Neither?
- What things do you believe in that give meaning to your life?
- What is your faith or belief?

I: Importance and Influence of Beliefs
Specific questions to elicit responses:
- Is your faith or belief important in your life?
- What influence does your faith or belief have on how you take care of yourself?
- How have your beliefs influenced your behavior during this illness?
- What role do your beliefs play in regaining your health?

C: Community
Specific questions to elicit responses:
- Are you part of a spiritual or religious community?
- Does the community provide support for you? How?
- Is there a person or group of people you really love or who are really important to you?

A: Address Care Issues
Specific question to elicit responses:
- How would you like me, as your healthcare provider, to address these issues while caring for you?

---

recognize their concerns as being "spiritual." The FICA tool was designed to be used in a time-constrained setting such as a routine visit, in which 2 minutes may be the only time allotted for a spiritual history.

Steinhauser demonstrated the validity of asking about "being at peace" when addressing spiritual contentment. Participants answered a question about the extent to which they felt "at peace." The trial involved 248 patients with terminal cancer, chronic obstructive pulmonary disease, and congestive heart failure, concluding that feeling at peace was strongly correlated with emotional and spiritual well-being in both traditional and nontraditional aspects of spirituality.[108]

Other spiritual tools include the brief version of the religious coping scale developed by Pargament and the Spiritual Well-Being Scale (SWBS). The Brief Religious Coping Scale (BRCOPE) has 14 items and measures positive and negative coping. The SWBS has 20 items and measures existential and spiritual well-being.

Interventions

The basic goal of intervention is to alleviate suffering by helping patients and families develop a sense of meaning that allows them to transcend their current situation. Spiritual healing is often possible when sources of pain are identified and specific interventions are applied. Although attention has been given to the importance of spiritual issues and the benefits of group therapy for existential pain, few interventions have been undertaken and studied specifically to alleviate spiritual pain. One trial evaluated the effect of the Supportive-Affective Group Experience for Persons with Life-Threatening Illness. Participants attended regular group sessions that focused on psychosocial and spiritual issues. The study was limited by its small size but showed positive effects on depressive symptoms, spiritual well-being, and a death-related loss of meaning.[109]

It is important to remember that interventions for relieving spiritual pain are rarely precise or orderly. The process of spiritual healing may require weeks, months, or even years, particularly after a series of especially traumatic events. When faced with a patient's deeply troubling spiritual pain, clinicians are likely to experience an initial sense of dismay and helplessness. However, it is from this sense of helplessness that physicians find a way to offer effective spiritual support.

The following interventions can help alleviate spiritual pain[110]:

- Listen to the patient's history. Be open to discussing painful issues. People often use alcohol, prescription drugs, and overactivity to avoid thinking about guilt, remorse, and other painful issues. When profound illness strikes, these methods of avoidance may no longer be possible. Painful and long-repressed thoughts may intrude and cause suffering. If guilt focuses on specific actions, emphasize atonement and forgiveness instead of trivializing the guilt by making statements such as "You shouldn't feel that way."

- Learn the patient's meaning system. (For more information, see "Reconstructing Meaning" on page 22 and Table 30 on page 58.)
- Listen with empathy. Acknowledge the difficulty of coping with unanswerable questions, particularly when so much of medicine involves the resolution of problems with technology and practical skill. Acknowledge the mystery of spirituality and resist the temptation to explain death or attach the patient's spiritual pain to religious doctrine.
- Help patients and family members formulate spiritual questions. Remember that exploring spiritual issues can be healing, even when no specific answers are revealed. Regardless of specific beliefs, a physician's continued presence and caring is paramount.
- Involve chaplains in pastoral care. Chaplains are consistently underused members of an interdisciplinary care team. (For more information, see UNIPAC 5.)
- Involve other interdisciplinary team members. Therapists can use interventions such as art, music, books, poetry, massage, prayer, meditation, and relaxation exercises to help patients access a sense of peace and unity and lessen the significance of remorse about the past, concerns about the future, and less-than-perfect systems of meaning.
- Provide information and improve communication. (For more information on communication, see UNIPAC 5.)
- Understand the dynamics of loss and grief. (See the chapter "Psychological Pain," pages 25 to 46.)
- Develop a spiritual and affective side. (See Table 28 on page 53 for more information.)

CLINICAL SITUATION

Sarah

Sarah is a 53-year-old woman with advanced breast cancer that has spread to her liver and brain. During the past year Sarah has undergone surgery and several courses of chemotherapy and radiation, but her disease is aggressive and relentless. During this hospital stay, Sarah's anger and impatience have irritated the entire hospital staff and driven away all her friends.

Because further curative treatment is no longer appropriate, Sarah is referred for hospice and palliative care. She will be transferred from the hospital to a hospice inpatient unit because her pain is difficult to control, she is extremely debilitated, and she has no one to care for her at home. The afternoon before Sarah's transfer to the hospice unit, her physician (who is feeling somewhat helpless because nothing can be done to slow Sarah's cancer) stops by to visit with Sarah. As soon as the physician walks in the room, Sarah expresses her anger about the upcoming transfer to the hospice inpatient unit and blames the physician for her progressive disease.

Question One

What is the physician's most appropriate course of action?
A. Leave the room until Sarah calms down and can discuss her situation rationally.
B. Cancel the referral for hospice and palliative care and order diazepam.
C. Sit down and listen to Sarah.
D. Educate Sarah about the natural progression of aggressive cancer.

Correct Response and Analysis

A is incorrect; leaving the room is a rejection of a patient's feelings, and Sarah has every reason to be upset about her condition. B is incorrect because canceling the referral and tranquilizing Sarah will not resolve her fears.

C is the correct response. The physician should recognize that Sarah's anger is probably caused by fear. By simply sitting down and listening, the physician can help reestablish Sarah's feelings of value and self-worth. Careful listening is also likely to elicit information that will be helpful when planning interventions to relieve Sarah's total pain.

D is incorrect because Sarah does not need information at this time; instead, she needs empathetic presence and the opportunity to express her fears to someone who can listen without judgment. In any case, until her fear and anger subside, Sarah will not be able to hear any important information.

The Case Continues

The physician sits at Sarah's bedside, leans toward her, and exhibits empathy by verbally recognizing her painful and difficult situation. The physician then asks Sarah to describe the main events that are causing her pain and anger. At first Sarah cries, but then she talks about the isolation she has experienced since her husband's death. She mentions that she stopped going to her synagogue shortly after her husband died because she was angry at the congregation, which was not supportive enough during her time of grief. Sarah also talks about her only child, a 22-year-old son, who experienced a difficult adolescence and has been alienated from Sarah for several years.

After acknowledging the pain these events have caused, the physician asks Sarah about any physical pain she is experiencing. Sarah indicates she still has quite a bit of pain but says it is somewhat improved.

Question Two

What is an appropriate course of action for the physician? (Select all that apply.)

A. Tell Sarah the visit must end because other patients are waiting and there is not enough time to address her concerns now.

B. Ask Sarah if she would like to see a rabbi.

C. Ask Sarah to describe her physical symptoms more carefully.

D. Tell Sarah to wait until the next day, when the hospice program will solve her problems.

Correct Responses and Analysis

A is incorrect because Sarah's suffering needs to be addressed, and it is likely that arranging for effective interventions will take much more time.

B and C are the correct responses. Physical and spiritual pain are significant contributors to suffering, and Sarah is clearly suffering. Her lingering physical pain and the spiritual pain she indicated when describing her alienation from the synagogue should be addressed as soon as possible.

D is incorrect because a patient should not have to wait to be transferred to a hospice and palliative inpatient unit before receiving relief from physical and spiritual pain.

The Case Concludes

When describing her pain, Sarah says it is deep, aching, and worsens on movement, which is consistent with soft-tissue and bone pain. The physician increases her dose of sustained-release morphine from 30 mg every 8 hours to 60 mg every 12 hours, with 10 mg of immediate-release morphine for breakthrough pain, and increases her dose of ibuprofen from 200 mg every 8 hours to 400 mg every 8 hours. Then, with Sarah's permission, the physician asks the chaplain to call a community rabbi and arrange for the rabbi to visit with Sarah later that evening. Before visiting, the rabbi confers with the social worker regarding existing plans of care and issues related to Sarah's son.

When the rabbi arrives, they discuss Sarah's spiritual concerns and the religious rituals that were meaningful to her in the past. Because Hanukkah is approaching, the rabbi lights candles on the electric menorah used for hospital visits, and together they recite traditional prayers for hope, healing, and forgiveness. Sarah is deeply moved and cries throughout the ceremony. Later she says the religious rituals helped her feel reconnected to her faith.

After Sarah is transferred to the hospice and palliative care inpatient unit, the rabbi continues to visit. With Sarah's permission, the hospice social worker arranges for Sarah's son to visit and, during their time together, Sarah and her son are able to forgive many of their past hurts and begin saying their goodbyes.

During Sarah's stay in the inpatient unit, the staff perceives her as kind, good-humored, pleasant to visit, and appreciative of their efforts to keep her comfortable. Sarah's pain becomes easier to manage and, when her physician visits, Sarah describes the transition from the hospital to the hospice inpatient unit as one of death and rebirth. She says she has been able to let go of much of her anger and has developed a new appreciation for being alive. She indicates the rabbi's visits are very meaningful and have been a major part of her healing. Sarah dies quietly a few days later.

Major World Religions and Their Frameworks

Cultures develop rituals that teach people how to act in situations that vary from greeting a friend to saying goodbye to someone who is dying.[111] To help make sense of the mystery of death and help mourners with the bereavement process, most religions emphasize the sacredness of dying and interpret it as an opportunity to connect with life's ultimate meaning and purpose. The death-related beliefs and rituals of many religions focus on the impermanence of life and the existence of an ultimate reality that transcends death.[112]

Because a patient's religious beliefs about suffering, death, and the afterlife affect decisions about end-of-life care and events surrounding the dying process, physicians should understand the basic beliefs of the world's major religions and their likely impact on end-of-life care.[113] It is important to remember, however, that generalizations about any religion are problematic. Religious beliefs evolve continuously to meet changing cultural conditions. Wide variations in beliefs and practices exist among practitioners of each of the world's religions.[114]

Because variations in belief occur even within specific religious subgroups, the best way to assess the likely impact of a patient's religious beliefs is to ask both the patient and the family. Physicians should never make assumptions based on community beliefs and traditions. The importance of addressing the issue of spirituality is evident in a Gallup survey, which demonstrated that 94% of polled Americans believe in God or a higher power and 60% stated that religion is an important aspect of their lives.[114] Patients and families should be offered the support of their community from chaplains and religious leaders.

Three major schools of thought surrounding religion and spirituality exist[115]:
- Theism—the belief in the existence of God (a supreme being), an immortal soul, or any other type of deity or deities.
- Atheism—the belief in the nonexistence of God or any type of supreme being or deity. Often associated with a materialist hypothesis that reality is defined through concrete matter.

- Agnosticism—the belief that the question of whether a supreme being exists cannot be answered or remains to be answered.

Death and the Afterlife

Most world religions view death as both an ending and a beginning—an end of life as it is currently known and the beginning of a new type of existence. In addition to the basic concepts of life after death that are listed below, an extraordinary number of individual beliefs exist concerning death and the afterlife.[114] This emphasizes the importance of addressing patient spirituality.

Heaven and Hell

The concept of a heaven and a hell is a characteristic of three major world religions: Judaism, Christianity, and Islam. According to these systems of belief, each human being lives a single life and, after death, survives as a disembodied soul. At some future date, the soul is reembodied and undergoes a last judgment by God, after which it enjoys eternal physical bliss in heaven or endures eternal physical anguish in hell. Many individual differences in interpretation exist, and belief in the actual existence of heaven and hell may be less common now than it was in the past.

Hope

The word "hope" is often a topic of discussion among a patient's family and healthcare providers. It can be used in the extreme setting of believing in irrational miracles and treatments. Conversations are often curtailed at the fear of taking away a person's hope. Judeo-Christian teachings emphasize we should not rely on miracles.[116] Biblical texts address hope and the comfort of prayer. Patients and families should never be made to feel there is nothing to hope for. Hope exists for relief of symptoms, comfort, reconciliation, and forgiveness. For more about hope, see page 13.

Forgiveness

The concept of forgiveness is pervasive in the teachings of Christianity. The ability to forgive is often coupled with the ability to understand and heal. Judaism and Islam also encourage forgiveness. In Judaism, forgiveness is earned through recognition and a commitment to abandon previous actions. Islam believes in the power of faith and forgiveness. Although the evidence is somewhat sparse, forgiveness may be associated with improved physical and mental health. Forgiveness is linked with reduced depression and anxiety.[117]

Rebirth

Although specific details differ, the Hindu and Buddhist traditions believe in a process of continuous rebirth, or reincarnation, until a state of oneness with ultimate reality is achieved. Then the process of rebirth ceases. The circumstances of reincarnation vary depending on karmic principles, such as the person's actions in a previous life. Belief in rebirth has become popular in the United States, even among some Christians.

CLINICAL SITUATION

Jim

Jim is a 26-year-old homosexual male with end-stage HIV/AIDS that is no longer responding to highly active antiretroviral therapy. He has been admitted to hospice home care with multiple infections that are not responding to treatment. He is experiencing shortness of breath and burning pain in his feet. Jim has several reliable caregivers, including his partner, his mother, and his sister. However, if his symptoms cannot be controlled at home, he will be transferred to hospice inpatient care.

During the physician's home visit, Jim is restless, cries easily, and looks generally miserable. The physician reads in the chart that Jim initially refused a visit from the hospice chaplain. While assessing for other sources of pain, the physician asks Jim if he would like to visit with the hospice chaplain. Jim gathers up his energy and yells, "Hell no!"

Question One

Which of the following are the physician's most appropriate courses of action? (Select all that apply.)

A. Note that Jim is likely to be experiencing spiritual pain.
B. Tell Jim not to swear.
C. Initiate intensive measures to relieve Jim's neuropathic pain and breathlessness.
D. Ask the chaplain to visit with Jim.

Correct Response and Analysis

Answers A and C are correct. Jim's response when offered a visit from the chaplain indicates that spiritual pain is most likely present. This should be discussed with the team and reassessed as soon as Jim's neuropathic pain and shortness of breath are alleviated.

B is incorrect because Jim's swearing is unlikely to harm anyone, and D is incorrect because it is contrary to the patient's stated wishes.

The Case Continues

The physician orders nortriptyline, 25 mg at bedtime, and valproate, 250 mg three times a day, to relieve the burning, stabbing sensations associated with neuropathic pain; oral morphine, 10 mg every 4 hours, is also ordered to help relieve Jim's neuropathic pain and shortness of breath.

Later the hospice nurse reports that these measures have greatly relieved Jim's physical discomfort, but his restlessness has increased and he looks even more miserable. During a subsequent visit, the physician and the medical social worker inquire about other sources of pain. Jim begins to cry and says he is afraid of dying. On further inquiry, Jim says he attended church regularly while he was growing up, but religious doctrines concerning homosexuality and attitudes about AIDS left him feeling hurt and abandoned, so he left the church.

Question Two

Which of the following interventions is most appropriate?

A. Tell Jim about the hospice program's nonjudgmental views about sexual orientation, encourage him to visit with the chaplain, and offer visits from a volunteer.
B. Denounce Jim's church for its lack of understanding.
C. Do not mention the chaplain again because Jim has already voiced his opposition.
D. Take time to personally help Jim with his spiritual pain, even though several other patients need to be seen and the physician is feeling very stressed.

Correct Response and Analysis

A is the correct response. The hospice philosophy of care, which promotes acceptance of patients regardless of sexual orientation, may help restore Jim's sense of value and self-worth. Visits with the chaplain may help reduce his obvious spiritual pain.

B is incorrect because denouncing Jim's church will not help with his search for spiritual peace. C is incorrect because the situation has changed; now that Jim's physical pain is better controlled, he is more likely to be able to address his spiritual needs. Continuing reassessment of all types of pain is appropriate. Offering interventions that initially were refused provides the patient with an opportunity to change directions and try something new.

D is incorrect because scheduling pressures and the physician's own stress are likely to lessen the quality of the intervention. Instead, involving other team members, such as the chaplain, medical social worker, and a volunteer, is more likely to deliver the intensive spiritual interventions he needs. If Jim does not feel comfortable talking to the chaplain or other counselors, the physician can schedule a visit with Jim for a less busy time.

The Case Concludes

During the course of many visits with an experienced, skilled hospice chaplain, Jim is finally able to tell his entire life story to a nonjudgmental listener. He experiences forgiveness when the chaplain asks him to forgive the church for the harm it did to him. As Jim's spiritual distress subsides, his neuropathic pain and shortness of breath are easier to control and his demeanor is more relaxed. Members of the hospice team are surprised by the changes in Jim and are even more surprised when he asks a volunteer to read scriptures to him. Jim requests audiotapes of spiritual music, and he dies calmly at home several weeks later, surrounded by family, friends, and hospice volunteers.

Faith Traditions and Hospice and Palliative Care

The beliefs of most of the world's major faiths are consistent with the goals and practices of hospice and palliative care, which are focusing care on the treatment of symptoms when a cure is no longer possible, alleviating pain even though it may result in sedation, and caring for all dimensions of the person—physical, emotional, social, and spiritual.

The most conservative branches of some religions may be less accepting of hospice and palliative care because of beliefs that life must be prolonged regardless of its quality or the likely burdens of treatment and that adequate measures to control severe pain must be resisted because they might shorten life for even a few hours. These religions believe physical suffering is necessary for spiritual development and must be endured.[113]

Religious Frameworks of Meaning

All cultures have developed systems of belief, rituals, and stories that provide a framework for making sense of life, death, and suffering. Eastern religions such as Hinduism and Buddhism view the material world as an illusion. In general, the spiritual goal is release from the suffering caused by worldly illusions and eventual union with a selfless and eternal bliss. Judaism, Christianity, and Islam view the material world as an important creation of God. In general, the spiritual goal is righteous living on Earth and eventual individual union with God in eternal bliss. Unlike

Hinduism, Buddhism, and Judaism, Christianity and Islam require a belief in specific religious doctrines.

Unless otherwise noted, the following descriptions of the basic beliefs of Hinduism, Buddhism, Judaism, Christianity, and Islam are based primarily on Houston Smith's book *The World Religions: Our Great Wisdom Traditions.*[111]

Hinduism

Hinduism, the religion of more than 730 million people,[118] is an amalgam of traditions, rituals, devotions, and philosophical systems developed over the past 4,500 years. Although polytheism is the basis for much popular Hindu worship, Hindus believe in the essential oneness of ultimate reality.

Hindus believe humanity's perception of the world as a multitude of differences is an illusion. Instead, they believe that ultimate reality, referred to as Brahman, is eternal oneness. Spiritual practices, such as yoga, focus on developing selflessness and transforming awareness. Such practices help dispel worldly illusions, leading to blissful union with Brahman (which means "God" in Sanskrit). Most Hindus believe they will endure many incarnations before attaining union with Brahman; however, some sects believe a gracious divinity such as Vishnu will help them achieve union more quickly.

Suffering

According to Hindu beliefs, there are three main causes of suffering. First is physical and psychological pain, which can be alleviated by using medications, reducing the fear that usually accompanies pain, and changing perspective from one that is limited and personal to one that approximates a larger, God's-eye view. Second is ignorance, which can be alleviated with education and increased insight. And third is a restricted sense of being, which can be alleviated by realizing that an eternal self (called Atman) underlies the human self and is actually a part of ultimate reality. Hindu scriptures, including the Vedas and the Bhagavad Gita, focus on achieving awareness of the eternal self and on attaining union with Brahman.

Death

For Hindus, death is natural and unavoidable, but it is not actually real. Only Brahman and Atman are ultimately real. As death approaches, religious rites and ceremonies provide support for the dying person. Traditionally, a son or relative puts water from the Ganges River in the dying person's mouth to bring peace and comfort. Family members and friends sing devotional prayers, read Hindu scriptures, and recite mantras to reassure the dying person with comforting words and the gentle tones of chanting. After death occurs, the body is washed, anointed, and dressed in new clothes, and the hair and beard are trimmed. Most Hindus believe cremation offers the best way for the soul to begin its journey.[112]

Implications for Hospice and Palliative Care

Most Hindus do not eat beef and may be strict vegetarians. Hindus often practice regular fasting, which can affect pain and symptom control measures as the intake of food and fluids is restricted. Physical cleanliness and modesty are of great concern.[119] Because bathing is viewed as both physically and spiritually cleansing, Hindu patients usually want to bathe daily in running water, a requirement that hospice and palliative care programs should strive to meet as a way of supporting the patient's spiritual needs. The Hindu emphasis on modesty can affect physical examinations, discussions of genitourinary and bowel functioning, and bed baths. Hindu patients generally prefer physicians and nurses of their own gender. The use of traditional Hindu (ayurvedic) medicine should be respected and combined with Western treatments, when possible.

Buddhism

Buddhism is the religious and philosophical system of more than 300 million people worldwide.[118] Buddhism is based on the teachings of Gautama Buddha, who lived in the sixth century BCE. Buddha resisted his followers' attempts to deify him. Instead, he encouraged people to focus on living ethically in this world and achieving enlightenment rather than focusing on the nature of God or the afterlife, both of which are inconceivable to the human mind.

Buddhism focuses on the search for awareness and the attainment of unconditional and selfless compassion. Buddhists believe it is possible to achieve enlightenment and enter nirvana by abandoning desires and delusions. Nirvana is described as incomprehensible and blissful liberation from suffering and release from reincarnation.

Suffering

Buddhism is based on Hinduism, but it rejects certain features of Hinduism, in particular the caste system. Buddhism recognizes Four Noble Truths:
1. Life is essentially suffering or dissatisfaction.
2. The origin of suffering lies in attachments, craving pleasure, and resisting painful experiences.
3. The cessation of suffering is possible by letting go of attachments, cravings, and resistance.
4. The way to cease craving and escape from continual rebirth is to follow the Buddhist practices known as the Noble Eightfold Path.

According to Buddhist beliefs, suffering results from ignorance, selfish desires, and attachment to the illusions of this world. Relief from suffering can be achieved by following the Noble Eightfold Path.

Buddhist Noble Eightfold Path

1. *Right views.* Use the resources of the mind and its intellectual orientation to examine life's problems. Ignorance is the primary cause of suffering, and life's greatest ignorance is the belief that people can imagine their final destiny.
2. *Right intent.* Persist in attempts to achieve awareness and enlightenment.
3. *Right speech.* Practice kindness and truth.
4. *Right conduct.* Refrain from killing, stealing, lying, drinking intoxicants, and sexual immorality.
5. *Right livelihood.* Engage in occupations that promote oneness instead of destroying it.
6. *Right effort.* Use the individual will to persevere toward the goal of enlightenment.
7. *Right mindfulness.* Continue self-examination to understand the self and see life as it really is.
8. *Right concentration.* Meditate, contemplate, and practice yoga.

Death

Unlike Hindus, who reject immortality of the body but believe that an eternal soul, or Self, transmigrates from one reincarnation to another, Buddhists believe in reincar-nation but reject immortality of both the body and soul. According to Buddhist belief (there are many variations), when death occurs, the temporarily bonded materials that compose human beings—matter, sensations, perceptions, mental formations, and consciousness—dissolve, but the life stream continues, even though no underlying self or permanent entity migrates to the next reincarnation. Buddhist beliefs about dying and rebirth are often compared to a candle flame; when the flame touches the wick of an unlighted candle, the light passes from one candle to another, even though the actual flame of the first candle does not pass over to the second candle.

Although Buddhist death practices vary greatly from country to country, there is general agreement that a dying person's state of mind is of great importance.[112] To help the patient achieve peace of mind, family, friends, and monks often surround the dying person, read religious texts, and repeat mantras. After death occurs, the body is washed, dressed in burial clothes, and cremated. Some Buddhists believe the dead person's conscious soul remains in or around the body for several days; monks are invited to chant sacred texts to assist the dead person's passage to the spiritual world and relieve the mourners' fears.

Implications for Hospice and Palliative Care

Although specific religious practices vary depending on local culture, the search for awareness is central to Buddhism, which means that Buddhists may be reluctant to use drugs that interfere with the practice of meditation. For some Buddhists, the spiritual pain resulting from an inability to meditate, whether due to a noisy environment or medication, may cause more suffering than uncontrolled physical pain.[119] Hospice and palliative care staff may have difficulty accepting a religious practice that prohibits the use of pharmacological therapies. However, other Buddhists seek symptom control because it enhances their ability to focus on peaceful calming of their spirit instead of on bodily distress.

Buddhists tend to be strict vegetarians and, like Hindus, often place high value on modesty and personal hygiene. Female patients may prefer to be cared for by female physicians and nurses. Buddhist families often ask that a patient's corpse remain untouched for as long as possible after death so its spirit can make a peaceful transition to the next world.

Judaism

Judaism is the religion of more than 17 million people worldwide.[118] It is based on the belief in one eternal God who created the universe, is omnipotent and all knowing, and communicates with human beings through revelation. Throughout their nearly 3,000-year history, the followers of Judaism have engaged in a passionate search for meaning and rely heavily on the five books of the Torah for spiritual authority and inspiration.[120]

The Torah, a collection of books written over a period of almost 1,000 years, is essentially a narrative history of the Jewish people's attempts to understand God's actions on Earth and to determine his will.[114] A particular scripture of the Torah is recited daily and includes divine instructions for living a righteous life.

Throughout much of their history, Jews have lived in exile and endured persecution, experiences that contribute to their exceptionally strong affirmation of the importance of life and family, observing traditional religious rituals, and obeying God's laws as described in the Torah.

Jewish tradition sanctifies everyday aspects of life with traditional rites and rituals embodying the spiritual meaning of both everyday and historic events. According to Jewish belief, even the smallest element of life, if rightly approached, is a reflection of God's infinite holiness.

Judaism views the world as good because it was created by God. Jews are expected to enjoy the bounty of this world, express their gratitude to God, and use the world's gifts for the betterment of humankind and the service of God. According to Jewish belief, people do not inherit original sin; they are born with a propensity for both good and evil and are responsible for their own actions.

Suffering

In general, suffering results from disobedience of God's laws as described in the Torah. Relief from suffering is possible by asking for God's forgiveness, living in accordance with God's divine will, bearing witness to God's purpose in the world, and living righteously in a way that improves the social order. When times of difficulty occur, Jews often draw spiritual nourishment, comfort, and meaning from scriptures, religious rituals, family relationships, and their history as a people.

Death

A wide range of beliefs concerning the afterlife exists within Judaism, from no specific view to a belief in the resurrection of the body and the immortality of the soul. In general, death is viewed as a necessary part of God's creation, not as a punishment for sin.

Some Jews, particularly those of Orthodox belief, hope for personal salvation and the coming of a Messiah who will usher in God's kingdom on Earth, at which time the bodies of the dead will be resurrected and rejoined with their souls. The righteous will then arise to be with God eternally and the wicked will be annihilated from memory.

Other Jews tend to view salvation more as an assurance of continued existence for the whole of creation rather than as eternal life for specific individuals. In any case, Judaism tends to focus on how life is lived on Earth rather than on events occurring after death, which are generally viewed as being more appropriately left to God.

According to Jewish belief, dying patients should be attended to almost constantly.[112] Family members and a rabbi frequently read from specific religious texts and recite psalms. Just before death occurs, the dying person is encouraged to make a confession, pray for forgiveness, and repeat specific prayers. From the time of death until the funeral, the body is rarely left unattended. Because most Jews do not believe in embalming or cremation, burial is encouraged within 24 hours of death.

At the end of the funeral service, relatives recite the Kaddish, a mourner's prayer, and often observe a prescribed 7-day period of mourning, during which they remain at home, recite evening prayers, and are comforted by visitors. Less rigorous mourning rituals are followed for up to 11 months after the funeral.

Implications for Hospice and Palliative Care

Because Judaism values life so highly, there was initial resistance to the concepts of hospice and palliative care within the Jewish community. The loss of even a few minutes of the precious gift of life was viewed as a terrible waste. As increasing evidence demonstrated that effective symptom control allowed dying patients to focus on spiritual concerns rather than physical pain, acceptance of palliative care increased.[119]

During a terminal illness, Jews often turn to traditional ritual observances for comfort and a sense of belonging. Caregivers can support the spiritual needs of Jewish patients by helping them observe days of special religious significance, including the Sabbath. Sabbath begins at sundown on Friday with the lighting of candles and lasts until sundown on Saturday, when the candles are extinguished. In addition to observing holy days, many Jews observe strict dietary laws that prohibit pork and shellfish. Some Jews require that food be prepared according to kosher techniques (eg, different sets of cookware for meat and milk products). More stringent requirements regarding food preparation are often followed on holy days, particularly Passover. Inpatient settings may need to obtain food from organizations specializing in the preparation of kosher foods. [119]

After the patient's death, a son or relative closes the corpse's eyes and mouth and washes and dresses the body, preferably in a white shroud. Very traditional Jews will have the body placed on the floor and will watch over it at all times. There is often a strong opposition to autopsies and organ donation. Burials often take place the following day after the death has occurred unless it is during Sabbath. [119]

Christianity

Christianity is the religion of approximately 1.8 billion people worldwide.[118] It is based on the life and teachings of Jesus, who was most likely born in Palestine around 4 BCE and crucified sometime between 29 and 33 CE. Jesus's teaching and healing career in Galilee lasted about 3 years. Christians worship Jesus as the Christ, God incarnate. The birth of Jesus, his life and teachings, and his crucifixion and bodily resurrection are described in the Christian Bible. The basic Christian message is one of God's love for humankind and humanity's need to develop selfless and unconditional love, both for God and for all other people. Some Christians interpret the Bible literally, viewing it is the highest authority for all matters of faith and theology.

As with other religions, Christian beliefs are very diverse, but Christianity's three most distinctive tenets are the Trinity, the Incarnation, and Atonement. Although various denominations interpret the tenets differently, in general the doctrine of the Trinity affirms that God is fully one but is also three (Father, Son, and Holy Spirit), meaning that God can be apprehended either directly or through the Son or the Holy Spirit; the doctrine of Incarnation affirms that Christ was both fully divine and fully human; and the doctrine of Atonement affirms God's vicarious assumption of humankind's sin through his son, Jesus, and Jesus's willingness to die as the ultimate form of atonement for humankind's sins.

Suffering

According to many Christians, suffering is caused by sin, broadly defined as actions and thoughts that result in a sense of estrangement from God. This suffering can result in a limited understanding of love, a sense of guilt, and the fear of death. Suffering is relieved by God's grace and the belief in the promise of eternal life.

Death

In general, Christianity suggests that death is a consequence of humankind's condition of original sin. Many Christians believe death results in a temporary separation of the body and soul. After Christ's second coming, the bodies of the dead will rise up and rejoin their souls for final judgment, after which the righteous will be sent to heaven, where they will enjoy eternal bliss, and the wicked will be sent to hell for eternal punishment.

Christian funeral practices vary from simple observances to elaborate rituals. The early Catholic church developed the sacrament of last rites (now called the anointment of the sick), which is usually accompanied by two other sacraments, confession and communion. These rites are intended to provide Catholics with the courage to die by reminding them of Christ's love and the promise of eternal life. During the anointment of the sick, Catholic priests pray and anoint patients with holy oils. As death approaches, prayers are offered for the person's soul.[112]

Implications for Hospice and Palliative Care

Christian attitudes toward suffering and death are based on Christ's death and resurrection. Some Christian denominations emphasize humankind's sinfulness and eternal suffering in hell for sinful behavior rather than the possibility of redemption and eternal reward in heaven. The emphasis on punishment may result in considerable fear of death among some Christians. Hospice and palliative care staff may need to reassure anxious patients by arranging for ritualized confession and reconciliation (for Catholics, this must be administered by a priest) and by reminding them of Christ's loving presence. Patients also may need reassurance from pastoral care staff that physical pain is not a punishment for sin; it results from physiological changes in the body.

Islam

Islam is one of the world's fastest-growing religions, with more than 970 million members worldwide.[118] The word Islam means both peace and surrender and refers to the peace that follows total surrender of one's life to the will of God. Islamic religious and social systems are based on the teachings of the prophet Muhammad, who lived from 570 to 632 CE. With some striking differences, the following theological concepts of Islam are very similar to those of Judaism and Christianity:

- One invisible and ultimate reality (God) exists that is all powerful but also compassionate and merciful.
- God created the world; therefore, it is real and significant rather than an illusion.
- Each person has a unique and immortal soul and is responsible for his or her actions while on Earth.
- After death, each soul is judged by God and enjoys either eternal bliss in heaven or endures eternal punishment in hell.

The followers of Islam view Muhammad as the last of God's chosen prophets (previous prophets include Abraham, Moses, Isaiah, and Jesus). Muhammad's military successes, administrative skills, and religious beliefs altered most of the Arabic world during his lifetime. Muhammad disagreed with the religious beliefs of many of his countrymen; he thought traditional Arab religions were idolatrous, Jews were reinterpreting the universal religion of Abraham into an exclusively nationalistic system, and Christians were subscribing to beliefs that compromised monotheism (eg, the Trinity and the Incarnation).

Islam emphasizes four points: the sole sovereignty of Allah (or God), the sinfulness of idolatry, the certainty of resurrection, and Muhammad's divine vocation as the prophet for Allah. As with other world religions, diversity of belief and practice is common among various sects of Islam; however, most Muslims belong to one of two main groups: the Sunnis or the Shi'ites.

The Koran is the holy book of Islam, and its importance to Muslims cannot be overemphasized. It is a collection of divine revelations delivered to Muhammad over the course of 23 years by the angel Gabriel. The Koran is viewed as the culmination of God's earlier revelations in the Hebrew and Christian Bibles and is believed by Muslims to contain the infallible and final words of God. In the Koran, God speaks in the first person, describing himself and reciting laws that include explicit instructions for achieving a righteous life. Muslims tend to interpret the Koran literally and believe it offers the highest authority for all matters of faith, theology, and law.

According to Islam, God revealed the truth of monotheism, the Ten Commandments, the Golden Rule, and the Five Pillars of Islam, which describe the righteous life. The following are the Five Pillars of Islam:

1. Confession of faith: "There is no God but Allah, and Muhammad is his prophet."
2. Muslims need constant prayer to keep life in perspective, which means praying five times a day: on rising, when the sun reaches its zenith, at the middle of the sun's decline, at sunset, and before retiring.
3. There must be charity toward the poor, exemplified by donating 2.5% of all one's holdings to the less fortunate.
4. There must be observance of Ramadan (Islam's holy month), during which able-bodied Muslims are required to fast from dawn until sundown.
5. Pilgrimage to Mecca is required at least once during a lifetime, which serves as a reminder of humanity's equality before God. During the pilgrimage, all distinctions of rank and hierarchy are prohibited.

Suffering

Suffering is caused by alienation from the will of Allah and is relieved by total surrender and commitment to his will as embodied in the Koran. For Muslims, spiritual life and social life are inseparable. Society is based on the teachings of the Koran.

Death

For Muslims, creation, death, and resurrection are sacred and inseparable. Because life is viewed as a time to prepare the soul for passing into life after death, struggling against death is viewed as resisting the will of Allah. The Koran describes a barrier separating the living from the dead, prohibiting reincarnation.

Like some Christians, Muslims view heaven as a place of physical delight and hell as a place of physical torment. According to Islam, on the final day of reckoning Allah will judge people according to their acts. Although individual salvation depends on each person's actions, repentance is possible, offering hope for redemption. The Koran recognizes that individuals have different abilities and various degrees of insight into the truth of Allah. People who live according to the truth (to the best of their ability) can attain a place in heaven; however, those who are acquainted with the truth of Islam and reject it have no hope for salvation.

Islamic death practices vary, but the dying person often wants to sit or lie turned toward Mecca.[112] No official last rites exist; however, family members usually repeat prayers, read Islamic scriptures, and encourage the patient to repeat the statement of faith. After death, the unwashed body is wrapped in a plain sheet, the face is bandaged to keep the mouth and eyes closed, and the feet are tied together. At the mosque or at home, the body is bathed, perfumed, wrapped in white cotton, and buried as soon as possible. Autopsies are strongly resisted.

Implications for Hospice and Palliative Care[119]

Islamic teachings view death as the will of Allah. Because Muslims believe that only other Muslims should touch the corpse, non-Muslims should put on rubber gloves before straightening the limbs and should also turn the corpse's head toward the right so it can be buried with the face turned toward Mecca. Muslims often follow rigid dietary guidelines and are required to wash specific parts of the body before each of the required five daily periods of prayer. Assisting with daily prayers and dietary and hygiene requirements is essential to providing spiritual support for Muslims.

Nonreligious Frameworks of Meaning

Existentialism and logotherapy are examples of nonreligious frameworks of meaning.

Existentialism

Although existentialism is sometimes confused with nihilism, they are not the same. The basic tenet of existentialism is individual responsibility while living an authentic life.[121]

In existentialism, suffering is caused by continuing to search for nonexistent ultimate meaning in the mysterious and indecipherable world of human existence and by failing to take responsibility for one's actions. Suffering is relieved by living an authentic life, which emphasizes personal responsibility for developing meaning through individual actions, beliefs, and involvement—not by relying on external standards of meaning. Caregivers can help relieve suffering by avoiding religious dogma and helping patients define their own personal sense of meaning. As with any patient, reviewing life often serves as an effective technique for helping existentialists recognize themes of courage and authenticity in their lives.

Logotherapy

Logotherapy is a psychoanalytic method developed by Victor Frankl, author of the book *Man's Search for Meaning*.[37] Suffering is caused by a sense of meaninglessness in life and death.

Logotherapy teaches that suffering can be relieved by developing a sense of purpose and wholeness through external achievement (creating a work of art or attaining a goal); internal experience, or fully experiencing an encounter with something or someone (satisfaction with work or a loving relationship with another person); and personal transformation (by turning personal tragedy into triumph through personal growth when faced with a fate that cannot be changed). For more information on helping patients achieve a sense of purpose and meaning, see the section "Reconstructing Meaning" on page 22.

Charles

Charles is a wealthy 48-year-old business executive who was energetic and somewhat driven prior to a grand mal seizure that occurred during a business meeting. Tests revealed an inoperable melanoma in Charles's brain. When his condition deteriorated, Charles was referred for hospice home care.

Shortly after Charles began hospice home care, the physician and hospice chaplain made a joint home visit to assess his condition. During the assessment, they heard in greater detail what had been reported by other team members: Charles rejected his childhood religious training at an early age and began practicing Buddhist meditation as a spiritual discipline during his college years. As Charles's career became more demanding, he gradually stopped meditating. Since the cancer diagnosis, Charles has been practicing both traditional and alternative treatments. However, he is becoming increasingly angry, discouraged, restless, and tearful because he believes he ought to be able to stop the cancer with positive thoughts and visualization techniques. The melanoma, however, continues to progress rapidly.

Question One

What is the most appropriate intervention?
A. Prescribe an antidepressant for Charles.
B. Tell Charles to stop the alternative practices because they are not working.
C. Without consulting Charles, ask a minister from Charles's childhood church to visit with him.
D. Inquire further about the sources of Charles's distress.

Correct Response and Analysis

A and B are incorrect responses because more information is needed before taking such actions. C is incorrect because it is premature and presumptuous; the physician has no way of knowing if Charles would like to see a minister unless a visit is discussed.

D is correct. Further inquiry may reveal additional causes of Charles's distress.

The Case Concludes

On further inquiry, the physician and the hospice chaplain learn that Charles is afraid he is not meditating correctly. Charles's expression brightens considerably when the chaplain offers to contact a meditation teacher.

During the course of several short visits, the meditation teacher leads Charles through a series of guided meditations that focus on spiritual healing instead of physical cure. The teacher also encourages Charles to practice meditations that will help him let go of his previous roles, expectations, and concepts of self.

As the weeks pass, Charles requires aggressive management of his symptoms, but his anger and anxiety lessen and he is able to let go of his identification with his personality. This enlarged framework of meaning helps him see his life in a new context. The hospice staff comment that they really enjoy their time with Charles and frequently find excuses to visit him. One month after admission to the hospice program, Charles dies quietly with a relaxed expression on his face.

Summary

Patients approaching the end of life often experience intense suffering. The concept of total pain (physical, social, psychological, and spiritual pain) helps describe suffering. The skills and resources of an interdisciplinary palliative care team are required to assess the various components of total pain and intervene to alleviate these symptoms. Successful interventions can be achieved through effective and compassionate communication, reconstructing meaning, and conserving dignity. Members of an interdisciplinary team need to provide an empathetic presence and foster hope for patients and families. Finally, caregivers and families should be screened for complicated grief syndromes, and appropriate counseling and interventions should be implemented.

The prevalence of mood disorders is high in patients with comorbidities who are approaching the end of life. Symptoms of anxiety and depression should be identified and multidisciplinary therapy provided. Special attention to geriatric depression and the potential for suicide can identify the patients at highest risk and provide them with appropriate help for their psychological suffering.

Spiritual care is vital to the care of the dying patient. The interdisciplinary team can encourage spirituality, communication, and the quest for meaning without making broad assumptions. Ultimately, patients must experience and work through their psychological and spiritual conflict. Physicians and other members of the healthcare team can help patients and families find peace and healing in the midst of dying. When an atmosphere of nonjudgmental presence and caring is established, patients and families can change in ways they never thought possible. Although an interdisciplinary team cannot cure a patient's suffering, they can provide the means to alleviate it.

References

1. Seneca. Quoted by: Saunders C. Spiritual pain. *J Palliat Care*. 1988;4(3):29-32.

2. Ventafridda V, Ripamonti C, Tamburini M, Cassileth RB, De Conno F. Unendurable symptoms as prognostic indicators of impending death in terminal cancer patients. *Eur J Cancer*. 1990;26(9):1000-1001.

3. Walke LM, Gallo WT, Tinetti ME, Fried TR. The burden of symptoms among community-dwelling older persons with advanced chronic disease. *Arch Intern Med*. 2004;164(21):2321-2324.

4. Mitka M. Suggestions for help when the end is near. *JAMA*. 2000;284(19): 2441-2442.

5. Abraham A, Kutner JS, Beaty B. Suffering at the end of life in the setting of low physical symptom distress. *J Palliat Med*. 2006;9(3):658-665.

6. Chochinov HM. Dying, dignity, and new horizons in palliative end-of-life care. *CA Cancer J Clin*. 2006;56(2):84-103.

7. Storey P. Symptom control in dying. In: Berger AM, Portenoy RK, Weissman, DE, eds. *Principles and Practices of Supportive Oncology*. Philadelphia, PA: Lippincott-Raven; 1998:741-748.

8. Cassell EJ. *The Nature of Suffering and the Goals of Medicine*. New York, NY: Oxford University Press; 1991:33-34.

9. Blinderman CD, Cherny NI. Existential issues do not necessarily result in existential suffering: lessons from cancer patients in Israel. *Palliat Med*. 2005;19(5):371-380.

10. Williams BR. Dying young, dying poor: a sociological examination of existential suffering among low-socioeconomic status patients. *J Palliat Med*. 2004;7(1):27-37.

11. Brody H. "My story is broken; can you help me fix it?" Medical ethics and the joint construction of narrative. *Lit Med*. 1994;13(1):79-92.

12. Baumeister RF. *Meanings of Life*. New York, NY: Guilford Press; 1991.

13. Gregory D, English JC. The myth of control: suffering in palliative care. *J Palliat Care*. 1994;10(2):18-22.

14. Breitbart W, Chochinov HM, Passik SD. Psychiatric symptoms in palliative medicine. In: Doyle D, Hanks G, Cherny N, Calman K, eds. *Oxford Textbook of Palliative Medicine*. 3rd ed. New York, NY: Oxford Univeristy Press; 2005:747.

15. Saunders CM. The challenge of terminal care. In: Symington T, Carter RL, eds. *Scientific Foundations of Oncology*. London: Heinemann; 1976:673-679.

16. Bakan D. *Disease, Pain and Sacrifice: Toward a Psychology of Suffering*. Boston, MA: Beacon Press; 1971. Cited by: Cassell EJ. The nature of suffering and the goals of medicine. *New Engl J Med*. 1982;306(11):639-645.

17. Terry W, Olson LG. Unobvious wounds: the suffering of hospice patients. *Intern Med J*. 2004;34(11):604-607.

18. Billings JA, Stoeckle JD. *The Clinical Encounter: A Guide to the Medical Interview and Case Presentation*. 2nd ed. St. Louis, MO: Mosby; 1999.

19. Harvey T. Who is the chaplain anyway? Philosophy and integration of hospice chaplaincy. *Am J Hosp Palliat Care*. 1996;13(5):41-43.

20. Byock IR. When suffering persists. *J Palliat Care*. 1994;10(2):8-13.

21. Steinhauser KE, Christakis NA, Clipp EC, McNeilly M, McIntyre L, Tulsky JA. Factors considered important at the end of life by patients, family, physicians, and other care providers. *JAMA*. 2000;284(19):2476-2482.

22. Herr K, Bjoro K, Decker S. Tools for assessment of pain in nonverbal older adults with dementia: a state-of-the-science review. *J Pain Symptom Manage*. 2006;31(2):170-192.

23. Morita T, Tei Y, Inoue S. Impaired communication capacity and agitated delirium in the final week of terminally ill cancer patients: prevalence and identification of research focus. *J Pain Symptom Manage*. 2003;26(3):827-834.

24. Kennett CE. Participation in a creative arts project can foster hope in a hospice day centre. *Palliat Med*. 2000;14(5):419-425.

25. Herth K. Fostering hope in terminally ill people. *J Adv Nurs*. 1990;15(11):1250-1259.

26. Block SD. Psychological issues in end-of-life care. *J Palliat Med*. 2006;9(3):751-772.

27. Kissane DW, Clarke DM, Street AF. Demoralization syndrome—a relevant psychiatric diagnosis for palliative care. *J Palliat Care.* 2001;17(1):12-21.

28. Hirai K, Morita T, Kashiwagi T. Professionally perceived effectiveness of psychosocial interventions for existential suffering of terminally ill cancer patients. *Palliat Med.* 2003;17(8):688-694.

29. Lynn J. Learning to care for people with chronic illness facing the end of life. *JAMA.* 2000;284(19):2508-2511.

30. Hallenbeck J. Cultural consideration of death and dying in America. Presented at: Academy of Hospice Physician Annual Meeting; June 1996; Snowbird, UT.

31. Byock IR. The nature of suffering and the nature of opportunity at the end of life. *Clin Geriatr Med.* 1996;12(2):237-252.

32. Levine S. *Who Dies?* New York, NY: Anchor Books; 1982.

33. Chochinov HM, Hack T, Hassard T, Kristjanson LJ, McClement S, Harlos M. Dignity therapy: a novel psychotherapeutic intervention for patients near the end of life. *J Clin Oncol.* 2005;23(24):5520-5525.

34. Chochinov HM, Hack T, McClement S, Kristjanson LJ, Harlos M. Dignity in the terminally ill: a developing empirical model. *Soc Sci Med.* 2002;54(3):433-443.

35. Chochinov HM, Hack T, Hassard T, et al: Dignity in the terminally ill: a cross-sectional cohort study. *Lancet.* 2002;360:2026-2030.

36. Tolstoy, L. *Tolstoy's Short Fiction.* Katz MR, ed. New York, NY: W.W. Norton; 1991.

37. Frankl VE. *Man's Search for Meaning.* New York, NY: Washington Square Press; 1985.

38. Cassem NH. The dying patient. In: Hackett TP, Cassem NH, eds. *Massachusetts General Hospital Handbook of General Psychiatry.* 2nd ed. Littleton, MA: PSG Publishing; 1987:332-352.

39. Lichter L, Mooney J, Boyd M. Biography as therapy. *Palliat Med.* 1993;7(2):133-137.

40. Zuckoff A, Shear K, Frank E, Daley DC, Seligman K, Silowash R. Treating complicated grief and substance use disorders: a pilot study. *J Subst Abuse Treat.* 2006;30(3):205-211.

41. Jacob SR. The grief experience of older women whose husbands had hospice care. *J Adv Nurs.* 1996;24(2):280-286.

42. Stroebe M, Schut H. The dual process model of coping with bereavement: rationale and description. *Death Studies.* 23(3):197-224.

43. Worden JW. *Grief Counseling and Grief Therapy: A Handbook for the Mental Health Practitioner.* 2nd ed. New York, NY: Springer Publishing; 1991.

44. Maciejewski PK, Zhang B, Block SD, Prigerson HG. An empirical examination of the stage theory of grief. *JAMA.* 2007;297(7):716-723.

45. Massie MJ, Gagnon P, Holland JC. Depression and suicide in patients with cancer. *J Pain Symptom Manage.* 1994;9(5):325-340.

46. Massie MJ, Shakin EJ. Management of depression and anxiety in cancer patients. In: Breitbart W, Holland J, eds. *Psychiatric Aspects of Symptom Management in Cancer Patients.* Washington, DC: American Psychiatric Press; 1993:1-21.

47. Holland JC, Morrow GR, Schmale A, et al. A randomized clinical trial of alprazolam versus progressive muscle relaxation in cancer patients with anxiety and depressive symptoms. *J Clin Oncol.* 1991;9(6):1004-1011.

48. Lamberg L. Treating depression in medical conditions may improve quality of life. *JAMA.* 1996;276(11):857-858.

49. Massie MJ, Holland JC. The cancer patient with pain: psychiatric complications and their management. *Med Clin North Am.* 1987;71(2):243-258. Cited by: Massie MJ, Gagnon P, Holland JC. Depression and suicide in patients with cancer. *J Pain Symptom Manage.* 1994;9(5):325-340.

50. Derogatis LR, Morrow GR, Fetting J, et al. The prevalence of psychiatric disorders among cancer patients. *JAMA.* 1983;249(6):751-757. In: Doyle D, Hanks G, Cherny N, Calman K, eds. *Oxford Textbook of Palliatve Medicine.* 3rd ed. New York, NY: Oxford University Press; 2005:747.

51. Massie MJ, Holland JC. Consultation and liaison issues in cancer care. *Psychiatr Med.* 1987;5(4):343-359. Cited by: Massie MJ, Shakin EJ. Management of depression and anxiety in cancer patients. In: Brietbart W, Holland J. *Psychiatric Aspects of Symptom Management in Cancer Patients.* Washington, DC: American Psychiatric Press; 1993.

52. Bukberg J, Penman D, Holland JC. Depression in hospitalized cancer patients. *Psychosom Med.* 1984;46(3):199-212.

53. Holland JC. Anxiety and cancer: the patient and the family. *J Clin Psychiatry.* 1989;50(suppl):20-25. Cited by: Breitbart W, Chochinov HM, Passik S. Psychiatric aspects of palliative care. In: Doyle D, Hanks GWC, MacDonald N, eds. *Oxford Textbook of Palliative Medicine.* New York, NY: Oxford University Press; 1993:609-626.

54. Bruera E, MacEachern T, Ripamonti C, Hanson J. Subcutaneous morphine for dyspnea in cancer patients. *Ann Intern Med.* 1993;119(9):906-907.

55. American Psychiatric Association. *Diagnostic and Statistical Manual of Mental Disorders Text Revision.* 4th edition. Arlington, VA: American Psychiatric Publishing, Inc.; 2000.

56. Breitbart W, Chochinov HM, Passik S. Psychiatric aspects of palliative care. In: Doyle D, Hanks G, MacDonald N, eds. *Oxford Textbook of Palliative Medicine.* 2nd ed. New York: Oxford University Press; 1998:934-954.

57. Bruera E, Portenoy RK, eds. *Topics in Palliative Care.* Vol 3. New York: Oxford University Press; 1998.

58. Porter MR, Musselman DL, McDaniel JS, Nemeroff CB. From sadness to major depression: assessment and management in patients with cancer. In: Portenoy RK, Bruera E. *Topics in Palliative Care.* Vol 3. New York, NY: Oxford University Press; 1998:191-212.

59. Periyakoil VS, Hallenbeck J. Identifying and managing preparatory grief and depression at the end of life. *Am Family Physician.* 2002;65(5):883-890.

60. Edelstein B, Kalish KD, Drozdick LW, McKee DR. Assessment of depression and bereavement in older adults. In: Lichtenberg PA, ed. *Handbook of Assessment in Clinical Gerontology.* New York, NY: John Wiley and Sons; 1999:11-58.

61. van der Lee ML, van der Bom JG, Swarte NB, Heintz AP, de Graeff A, van den Bout J. Euthanasia and depression: a prospective cohort study among terminally ill cancer patients. *J Clin Oncol.* 2005;23(27):6607-6612.

62. Emanuel EJ. Depression, euthanasia, and improving end-of-life care. *J Clin Oncol.* 2005;23(27):6456-6458.

63. Chochinov HM, Wilson KG, Enns M, Lander S. "Are you depressed?" Screening for depression in the terminally ill. *Am J Psychiatry.* 1997;154(5):674-676.

64. Irwin M, Artin KH, Oxmnan MN. Screening for depression in the older adult: criterion validity of the 10-item Center for Epidemiological Studies Depression Scale (CES-D). *Arch Intern Med.* 1999;159(15):1701-1704.

65. Lewinsohn PM, Seeley JR, Roberts RE, Allen NB. Center for Epidemiological Studies Depression Scale (CES-D) as a screening instrument for depression among community-residing older adults. *Psychol Aging.* 1997;12(2):277-287.

66. Radloff LS. The CES-D scale: a self-report depression scale for research in the general population. *Appl Psychol Meas.* 1977;1(3):385-401.

67. Brink TL, Yesavage JA, Lum O, Heersema P, Adey MB, Rose TL. Screening tests for geriatric depression. *Clin Gerontol.* 1982;1:37-44.

68. Sheikh JI, Yesavage JA. Geriatric Depression Scale (GDS): Recent evidence and development of a shorter version. In: Brink T, ed. *Clinical Gerontology: A Guide to Assessment and Intervention.* New York, NY: The Haworth Press; 1986:165-173.

69. Breitbart W, Passik SD. Psychological and psychiatric interventions in pain control. In: Doyle D, Hanks G, MacDonald N, eds., *Oxford Textbook of Palliative Medicine.* New York, NY: Oxford University Press; 1993:244-256.

70. Serby M, Yu M. Overview: depression in the elderly. *Mt Sinai J Med.* 2003;70(1):38-44.

71. Cherny NI, Coyle N, Foley KM. The treatment of suffering when patients request elective death. *J Palliat Care.* 1994;10(2):71-79.

72. Emanuel EJ, Fairclough DL, Emanuel LL. Attitudes and desires related to euthanasia and physician-assisted suicide among terminally ill patients and their caregivers. *JAMA.* 2000;284(19):2460-2468.

73. Physician-assisted death [position statement]. Glenview, IL: American Academy of Hospice and Palliative Medicine; 2007 February 14. Available at: http://www.aahpm.org/positions/suicide.html. Accessed March 17, 2008.

74. Greene WR, Davis WH. Titrated intravenous barbiturates in the control of symptoms in patients with terminal cancer. *South Med J.* 1991;84(3):332-337.

75. Truog RD, Berde CB, Mitchell C, Grier HE. Barbiturates in the care of the terminally ill. *N Engl J Med.* 1992;327(23):1678-1682.

76. Rabow MW, Hauser JM, Adams J. Supporting family caregivers at the end of life: "They don't know what they don't know." *JAMA*. 2004;291(4):483-491.

77. National Alliance for Caregiving and AARP. Caregiving in the U.S. www.caregiving.org/data/04finalreport.pdf. Accessed July 13, 2007.

78. Hebert RS, Schulz R. Caregiving at the end of life. *J Palliat Med*. 2006;9(5):1174-1187.

79. Pearlin L, Mullan J, Semple S, Skaff M. Caregiving and the stress process: an overview of concepts and their measures. *Gerontologist*. 1990;30:583-594.

80. Schulz R, Hebert RS, Dew MA, et al. Patient suffering and caregiver compassion: new opportunities for research, practice, and policy. *Gerontologist*. 2007;47(1):4-13.

81. Cameron JI, Franche RL, Cheung AM, Stewart DE. Lifestyle interference and emotional distress in family caregivers of advanced cancer patients. *Cancer*. 2002;94(2):521-527.

82. Salmon JR, Kwak J, Acquaviva KD, Brandt K, Egan KA. Transformative aspects of caregiving at life's end. *J Pain Symptom Manage*. 2005;29(2):121-129.

83. Hauser JM, Kramer BJ. Family caregivers in palliative care. *Clin Geriatr Med*. 2004;20(4):671-688.

84. Diwan S, Hougham GW, Sachs GA. Strain experienced by caregivers of dementia patients receiving palliative care: findings from the Palliative Excellence in Alzheimer Care Efforts (PEACE) Program. *J Palliat Med*. 2004;7(6):797-807.

85. Waldrop DP, Kramer BJ, Skretny JA, Milch RA, Finn W. Final transitions: family caregiving at the end of life. *J Palliat Med*. 2005;8(3):623-638.

86. Hebert RS, Dang Q, Schulz R. Religious beliefs and practices are associated with better mental health in family caregivers of patients with dementia: findings from the REACH study. *Am J Geriatr Psych*. 2007;15(4):292-300.

87. Showalter SE. Coping with losses. *Am J Hosp Palliat Care*. 1996;13(5):46-48.

88. Lazare A. Unresolved grief. In: Lazare A, ed. *Outpatient Psychiatry: Diagnosis and Treatment*. 2nd ed. Baltimore, MD: Wilkins and Wilkins; 1988.

89. Shear K, Shair H. Attachment, loss, and complicated grief. *Dev Psychobiol*. 2005;47(3):253-267.

90. Shear K, Frank E, Houck PR, Reynolds CF. Treatment of complicated grief: a randomized controlled trial. *JAMA*. 2005;293(21):2601-2608.

91. Bonanno GA. Loss, trauma, and human resilience: have we underestimated the human capacity to thrive after extremely aversive events? *Am Psychol*. 2004;59(1):20-28.

92. Goldstein J, Alter CL, Axelrod R. A psychoeducational bereavement-support group for families provided in an outpatient cancer center. *J Cancer Educ*. 1996;11(4):233-237.

93. Sherman DW, Ouellette S. Physicians reflect on their lived experiences in long-term AIDS care. *J Palliat Med*. 2000;3(3):275-286.

94. Moadel A, Morgan C, Fatone A, et al. Seeking meaning and hope: self-reported spiritual and existential needs among an ethnically diverse cancer patient population. *Psychooncology*. 1999;8(5):378-385.

95. Doyle D. Have we looked beyond the physical and psychosocial? *J Pain Symptom Manage*. 1992;7(5):302-311.

96. Sulmasy DP. Spiritual issues in the care of dying patients: "…It's ok between me and God." *JAMA*. 2006;296(11):1385-1392.

97. Hay MW. Principles in building spiritual assessment tools. *Am J Hosp Care*. 1989;6(5):25-31.

98. Kellehear A. Spirituality and palliative care: a model of needs. *Palliat Med*. 2000;14(2):149-155.

99. Sulmasy DP. A biopsychosocial-spiritual model for the care of patients at the end of life. *Gerontologist*. 2002;42(spec no 3):24-33.

100. Office of Minority Health & Health Disparities, Centers for Disease Control and Prevention. Black or African American Populations. Available at: www.cdc.gov/omhd/Populations/BAA/BAA.htm. Accessed March 17, 2008.

101. Bullock K. Promoting advance directives among African Americans: a faith-based model. *J Palliat Med*. 2006;9(1):183-195.

102. Fortin AH, Barnett KG. Medical school curricula in spirituality and medicine. *JAMA*. 2004;291(23):2883.

103. Astin JA, Harkness E, Ernst E. The efficacy of "distant healing": A systematic review of randomized trials. *Ann Intern Med*. 2000;132(11):903-910.

104. Sloan R, Bagiella E, Powell T. Religion, spirituality, and medicine. *Lancet*. 1999;353(9153):664-667.

105. Post SG, Puchalski CM, Larson DB. Physicians and patient spirituality: professional boundaries, competency, and ethics. *Ann Intern Med*. 2000;132(7):578-583.

106. Ehman JW, Ott BB, Short TH, Ciampa RC, Hansen-Flaschen J. Do patients want physicians to inquire about their spiritual or religious beliefs if they become gravely ill? *Arch Intern Med*. 1999;159(15):1803-1806.

107. Puchalski CM. Spiritual Assessment Tool. *Innovations in End-of-Life Care*. 1999;1(6):1-2. www2.edc.org/lastacts/archives/archivesNov99/assesstool.asp. Accessed July 13, 2007.

108. Steinhauser KE, Voils CI, Clipp EC, Bosworth HB, Christakis NA, Tulsky JA. "Are you at peace?" One item to probe spiritual concerns at the end of life. *Arch Intern Med*. 2006;166(1):101-105.

109. Miller DK, Chibnall JT, Videen SD, Duckro PN. Supportive-affective group experience for persons with life-threatening illness: reducing spiritual, psychological, and death-related distress in dying patients. *J Palliat Med*. 2005;8(2):333-343.

110. McCabe MJ. Clinical response to spiritual issues. In: Portenoy RK, Bruera E, eds. *Topics in Palliative Care*. Vol. 1. New York, NY: Oxford University Press; 1997:279-290.

111. Smith H. *The World's Religions: Our Great Wisdom Traditions*. New York, NY: Harper Collins; 1991.

112. Kramer K. *The Sacred Art of Dying: How World Religions Understand Death*. New York, NY: Paulist Press; 1988.

113. Hamel RP, Lysaught MT. Choosing palliative care: do religious beliefs make a difference? *J Palliat Care*. 1994;10(3):61-66.

114. Armstrong K. *A History of God*. New York, NY: Ballantine Books; 1994.

115. Miovic M. An introduction to spiritual psychology: overview of the literature, east and west. *Harv Rev Psychiatry*. 2004;12(2):105-115.

116. Puchalski CM, Dorff ED, Hendi IY: Spirituality, religion, and healing in palliative care. *Clin Geriatr Med*. 2004;20:689-714.

117. Lawler KA, Younger JW, Piferi RL, Jobe RL, Edmondson KA, Jones WH. The unique effects of forgiveness on health: an exploration of pathways. *J Behav Med*. 2005;28(2):157-167.

118. Markham IS. *A World Religions Reader*. Boston, MA: Blackwell; 1996.

119. Neuberger JA. Cultural issues in palliative care. In: Doyle D, Hanks GWC, MacDonald N, eds. *Oxford Textbook of Palliative Medicine*. New York, NY: Oxford University Press; 1993:507-513.

120. Parrinder G, ed. *World Religions: From Ancient History to the Present*. New York, NY: Facts on File; 1984.

121. Drabble M, ed. *The Oxford Companion to English Literature*. 5th ed. New York, NY: Oxford University Press; 1985.

Pretest Correct Answers

1.	B		20.	B
2.	B		21.	A
3.	C		22.	D
4.	D		23.	D
5.	C		24.	B
6.	B		25.	D
7.	C		26.	B
8.	A		27.	C
9.	B		28.	B
10.	C		29.	C
11.	C		30.	C
12.	B		31.	B
13.	B		32.	D
14.	C		33.	C
15.	A		34.	C
16.	D		35.	B
17.	B		36.	C
18.	C		37.	D
19.	B			

Posttest and Evaluation Instructions

The American Academy of Hospice and Palliative Medicine now provides real-time grading and a real-time certificate for completing this posttest and evaluation online. Some accrediting organizations may not accept the CME from the third edition of the UNIPAC series if you have already obtained CME for the previous edition of the same UNIPAC. For clarification, please contact your accrediting organization. To take the posttest and complete the evaluation form, visit www.aahpm.org/education and under the heading "Self-Study" click on the UNIPAC link.

After successfully completing the posttest, first time customers will be asked to register and returning customers will be asked to log in. The cost to process your test and issue your certificate is $60. You will be asked to provide your credit card information for this posttest at the time of registration. Your posttest results will instantly be available for review, and you will then be asked to complete an evaluation form. Immediately after completing the evaluation form, you will be able to print your certificate from your browser.

You must correctly answer 28 of 37 questions for UNIPAC 2. If needed, you may retake the posttest. Please complete the evaluation form that will appear on your screen after passing the examination.

Occasionally computers fail. You may wish to print the posttest questions, mark the answers on the printed copy, then transfer those answers to the computer when you're ready to submit the posttest for scoring.

AAHPM welcomes your feedback. Please send comments and suggestions about this book to info@aahpm.org.